Handbook of Spirituality and Worldview in Clinical Practice

Handbook of Spirituality and Worldview in Clinical Practice

Edited by

Allan M. Josephson, M.D.

John R. Peteet, M.D.

Washington, DC
London, England

Note: The authors have worked to ensure that all information in this book is accurate at the time of publication and consistent with general psychiatric and medical standards, and that information concerning drug dosages, schedules, and routes of administration is accurate at the time of publication and consistent with standards set by the U.S. Food and Drug Administration and the general medical community. As medical research and practice continue to advance, however, therapeutic standards may change. Moreover, specific situations may require a specific therapeutic response not included in this book. For these reasons and because human and mechanical errors sometimes occur, we recommend that readers follow the advice of physicians directly involved in their care or the care of a member of their family.

Books published by American Psychiatric Publishing, Inc., represent the views and opinions of the individual authors and do not necessarily represent the policies and opinions of APPI or the American Psychiatric Association.

Manufactured in the United States of America on acid-free paper
08 07 06 05 04   5 4 3 2 1
First Edition

Typeset in Adobe's Berkeley and Univers

American Psychiatric Publishing, Inc.
1000 Wilson Boulevard
Arlington, VA 22209-3901
www.appi.org

Library of Congress Cataloging-in-Publication Data
Handbook of spirituality and worldview in clinical practice / [edited by] Allan M.
   Josephson, John R. Peteet.—1st ed.
       p. ; cm.
   Includes bibliographical references and index.
   ISBN 1-58562-104-8 (pbk. : alk. paper)
       1. Psychotherapy patients—Religious life. 2. Psychotherapy—Religious aspects.
3. Spirituality. 4. Spiritual life. 5. Psychotherapist and patient. 6. Psychiatry and
religion. I. Josephson, Allan M., 1951– II. Peteet, John R., 1947–
   [DNLM: 1. Spirituality. 2. Mental Disorders—therapy. 3. Religion and Medicine.
WM 420 H23655 2004]
RC489.R46H365 2004
616.89′14—dc22

                                                                                    2004050258

British Library Cataloguing in Publication Data
A CIP record is available from the British Library.

Contents

PART I
Conceptual Foundation

1 Introduction: Definition and Significance of a Worldview . .3

Armand M. Nicholi Jr., M.D.

PART II
Clinical Foundations

2 Worldview in Psychiatric Assessment 15

Allan M. Josephson, M.D.
Irving S. Wiesner, M.D.

3 Worldview in Diagnosis and Case Formulation 31

Allan M. Josephson, M.D.
John R. Peteet, M.D.

4 Therapeutic Implications of Worldview 47

John R. Peteet, M.D.

PART III
Patients and Their Traditions

5 Protestant Christians. 63

Mark E. Servis, M.D.

PART IV
Worldview and Culture

Contributors

Yousef Abou-Allaban, M.D.
Medical Director, Boston Health Care, and Assistant Professor of Psychiatry, University of Massachusetts Medical School, Walpole, Massachusetts

Richard L. Grant, M.D.
Clinical Professor of Psychiatry and Family Medicine, University of Illinois College of Medicine, Peoria, Illinois

David Greenberg, M.A., M.B., B.Chir., M.R.C.Psych.
Director of Psychiatric Services, Herzog-Ezrath-Nashim Hospital, and Senior Lecturer in Psychiatry, Hadassah Medical School, Hebrew University, Jerusalem, Israel

Judith Moss Hughes, M.D.
Private Practice of General Psychiatry, Worcester, Massachusetts

Allan M. Josephson, M.D.
Chief Executive Officer, Bingham Child Guidance Center; Professor and Chief, Division of Child and Adolescent Psychiatry, Department of Psychiatry and Behavioral Sciences, University of Louisville, Louisville, Kentucky

Nalini V. Juthani, M.D.
Director of Psychiatric Education, Bronx Lebanon Hospital, Bronx, New York; Professor of Clinical Psychiatry, Albert Einstein College of Medicine, Bronx, New York

Armand M. Nicholi Jr., M.D.
Associate Clinical Professor of Psychiatry, Harvard Medical School; Attending Psychiatrist, Massachusetts General Hospital, Boston, Massachusetts

John R. Peteet, M.D.
Associate Professor of Psychiatry, Harvard Medical School; Clinical Director, Psychiatry, Adult Psychosocial Oncology, Dana-Farber Cancer Institute; Attending Psychiatrist, Brigham and Women's Hospital, Boston, Massachusetts

Syed Atezaz Saeed, M.D.
Professor and Chairman, Department of Psychiatric Medicine, The Brody School of Medicine, East Carolina University, Greenville, North Carolina

Mark E. Servis, M.D.
Associate Professor of Psychiatry, Residency Training Director and Vice Chair, Department of Psychiatry and Behavioral Science, University of California at Davis, Sacramento, California

Samuel B. Thielman, M.D., Ph.D.
Adjunct Assistant Professor, Department of Psychiatry and Behavioral Sciences, Duke University School of Medicine, Durham, North Carolina; Director, Mental Health Services, Office of Medical Services, U.S. Department of State, Washington, DC

Irving S. Wiesner, M.D.
Clinical Assistant Professor (Adjunct), Department of Psychiatry and Behavioral Sciences, Temple University School of Medicine; Private Practice of General Psychiatry, Swarthmore, Pennsylvania; Chair, Committee on Religion, Spirituality, and Psychiatry, American Psychiatric Association

Preface

This work began with questions that several of us had as we struggled to understand the place of our own and our patients' worldviews in our clinical work. Collaborative exploration of these issues among colleagues, several of whom have authored chapters in this volume, led to several presentations at annual meetings of the American Psychiatric Association. Over the past decade, these workshops, symposia, and courses have increasingly focused on the worldview of the clinician as an underappreciated variable in the clinical encounter. More recently they have also included presentations by psychiatrists who represent specific worldviews. This book is the published result of these activities.

Psychiatry has been undergoing rapid change in its relationship not only to the neurosciences but also to religion and spirituality. Clinicians increasingly recognize the importance of cultural differences and incorporate spiritual approaches into treatments of the various disorders that occur throughout the life span. A growing clinical literature discusses spirituality, and a developing research literature correlates measures of religion and health. Training requirements increasingly include experience in assessing and managing cultural, religious, and spiritual issues in clinical care.

Greater openness to considering religious and spiritual factors in mental health treatment has stimulated a number of intensely practical questions: How much should clinicians support the use of religious practices that appear to be therapeutic? What are the best ways to recognize and deal with religion's negative effects? What is the role of a therapist's own belief system in approaching these questions? In the past, mental health professionals have often avoided these questions, either actively as a choice or passively because of discomfort. Fortunately, several authors, including Richards and Bergin (1997), Koenig (1998), and Boehnlein (2000), have provided considerable background information for clinicians who work with individuals from various faith traditions. We hope that this volume adds to this literature in two ways.

First, in this book we offer a systematic framework for understanding the diagnostic and therapeutic implications of different systems of belief and apply this framework in the consideration of specific religious and spiritual traditions. We have included among these traditions the perspective of the atheistic or agnostic patient and clinician, something not typically done in previous works. This inclusion underscores a major theme of this work: worldview must be considered in all individuals, not just those from a formal religious or spiritual tradition. Everyone has a worldview, whether he or she realizes it or not.

Second, we have asked the contributing authors to emphasize the clinical problems that may be faced by persons with a particular tradition and not solely to describe elements of the faith itself. Hence the chapters are entitled, for example, "Jews," not "Judaism," and "Muslims," not "Islam." The book is not primarily about religion and spirituality but about patients and clinicians, the worldviews they possess, and how their worldviews affect their daily lives. This work also includes a discussion of practical approaches to clinical problems that present when patients and clinicians do or do not share the same worldview.

We have chosen to focus on belief to the relative neglect of practice, community, and experience. This approach seemed important because what people believe makes a difference in how they think, feel, and behave. Readers can find help in working with other aspects of faith by consulting works such as *Encountering the Sacred in Psychotherapy: How to Talk With People About Their Spiritual Lives* (Griffith and Griffith 2002). Several other principles undergird this work: that religion and spirituality are not cures for mental disorders but are usually pursued for their own purposes; that religion and spirituality can have positive and negative effects; and that the illness experience can lead individuals toward, or away from, a religious or spiritual approach to life.

We struggled with several challenges. The first set of challenges consisted of limiting, focusing, and defining this expansive topic. Space limitations forced the discussion of adherents to address only some of the traditions commonly encountered by Western clinicians: Protestant and Catholic Christians, Jews, Muslims, Hindus and Buddhists, and atheists and agnostics. We have not, for example, directly considered Latter Day Saints, Christian Scientists, Sikhs, adherents of traditional Native American religions, and believers in spiritism. Nor have we discussed the many individuals who hold tenets of more than one system of belief or who are unsure what they believe. We have also not been able to discuss extensively the differences within faiths (sects, divisions) that are extremely important to many of their adherents.

Using terms clearly was a second challenge. The definitions of religion and spirituality remain elusive, and our offerings are not the final answer. We see spirituality as concerned with one's connection to a larger context of meaning, and religion as the form that spirituality takes within given traditions. The less commonly used term *worldview* refers to an intellectual response to life's most basic questions (see Chapter 1, "Introduction: Definition and Significance of a Worldview") that is important to individuals whether or not they consider themselves spiritual or religious. Rather than focusing on the differences between spirituality, religion, and worldview, we have used the terms more or less interchangeably in the title and throughout the text.

We counted on chapter authors to use their knowledge as insiders to describe their respective traditions, but we also asked them to indicate the ways that beliefs within these traditions may sometimes be recruited to support psychopathology or may be held for dynamic reasons. Although we encouraged the authors to be dispassionate, at times their ardor shows through. We believe that this tendency underscores a central point of this volume: that everyone has a worldview and feels strongly about its truth. Finally, because this book is a clinical volume, we could make only indirect reference to research.

The book is organized into four sections: 1) an introduction to the concept of worldview and its significance; 2) chapters that address issues of general clinical significance, including assessment, formulation, and therapeutic implications of worldview; 3) a section that considers the clinical implications of several major traditions of belief; and 4) a concluding chapter that considers the large role played by culture in understanding the worldviews of others, particularly those living in or coming from a non-Western setting.

Each author in the third section followed a standard format of considering core beliefs and practices; diagnostic challenges and core therapeutic dilemmas presented by adherents; variations in clinical encounters, depending on whether the clinician and the patient share the same worldview; and opportunities for collaboration with outside resources, such as clergy or other religious or spiritual advisors.

Our hope is that in this compact volume we make clear how an understanding of our own and our patients' worldviews can enhance all clinical work. We envision this book as both a basic text for mental health professionals who are teaching in and learning about this emerging area and as a stimulus to explore the importance of worldview in greater depth.

Acknowledgments

We are grateful to numerous individuals for their contributions to this work:

- Leigh Bishop and Dan Blazer, who inspired us to ask larger questions;
- Roger Sider, whose ethical insights were invaluable and who hosted early attempts by a group of us to explore this area;
- Armand Nicholi, whose clarity of thought reminded us that everyone has a worldview;

- Irv Wiesner, who expanded our conversations to include psychiatrists committed to a wide variety of worldviews;
- All our contributing authors, who worked hard to fit their thoughts into our frame of reference;
- Mansell Pattison and David Larson, who early on challenged academic psychiatry to recognize the importance of faith;
- Bob Hales and John McDuffie, who guided this work to completion;
- The many others whose indirect contributions made this work possible, including Alan and Bev Bergstrom, Dick Bagge, Jeff Brandsma, Alex Mabe, Frank Moncher, Timothy Owings, Rodger Murchison, Neil Graham, Don Posterski, and Mary McCarthy;
- Finally, our parents Albert and Anna Josephson and Mary and Dennie Peteet, who introduced us to the relationship between faith and behavior, and our spouses Jeri and Jean, who generously gave us time and support.

Allan M. Josephson, M.D.
Louisville, Kentucky

John R. Peteet, M.D.
Boston, Massachusetts

References

Boehnlein JK: Psychiatry and Religion: The Convergence of Mind and Spirit. Washington, DC, American Psychiatric Press, 2000

Griffith JL, Griffith ME: Encountering the Sacred in Psychotherapy: How to Talk With People About Their Spiritual Lives. New York, Guilford, 2002

Koenig HG, Pritchett J: Religion and psychotherapy, in Handbook of Religion and Mental Health. Edited by Koenig HG. San Diego, CA, Academic Press, 1998, pp 323–336

Richards PS, Bergin A: A Spiritual Strategy for Counseling and Psychotherapy. Washington, DC, American Psychological Association, 1997

PART I

Conceptual Foundation

Introduction

Definition and Significance of a Worldview

Armand M. Nicholi Jr., M.D.

The concept of a worldview has profound implications for the clinician. The worldview of the patient as well as the worldview of the clinician contributes to the success or failure of the clinician-patient relationship. The key to understanding the patient rests heavily on understanding the patient's worldview. The worldview of the clinician may not only conflict with the patient's worldview but may also influence his or her clinical observations and clinical judgment.

How do we define worldview? What influences shape the development of one's worldview? In this introductory chapter, I consider these questions using the example of the life and work of Sigmund Freud.

Why Freud? No individual has influenced the field of psychiatry more profoundly than Freud, the father of psychoanalysis. His contributions form the basis of the most extensively developed theory of the mind. In addition, most psychodynamic psychotherapies use one or more of his concepts. Along with making these contributions, Freud helped to define the concept of a weltanschauung, or worldview. His relentless argument for a scientific (materialistic) worldview has caused Freud and psychiatry, until recently, to be seen by some as undermining spiritual values. Freud's biographers wrote extensively about the influences that shaped the development of his worldview.

Freud's life vividly demonstrates the significance of worldview and provides an implicit message for all clinicians—whether one realizes it or not, everyone possesses a worldview. Our worldview tells us more about ourselves than any other part of our personal history and influences how patients present to us and how we respond as clinicians.

Definition of Worldview

How does one define "worldview"? In 1933, Freud wrote "The Question of a Weltanschauung," the last of the New Introductory Lectures. He defined a weltanschauung (which, literally translated, means "view of the world") as "an intellectual construction which solves all the problems of our existence uniformly on the basis of one overriding hypothesis ..." (Freud 1933/1962, p. 158). As Freud described it, a weltanschauung is a philosophy of life that answers all of the most fundamental questions of human existence. He discussed at length what he called the "scientific" worldview and expended great time and energy comparing and contrasting this view with the spiritual worldview. The scientific worldview, Freud stated, precludes all knowledge of the universe "other than the intellectual working over of carefully scrutinized observations—in other words, what we call research" (Freud 1933/1962, p. 159).

Freud recognized that we all possess a worldview, and he divided people into two categories: believers and unbelievers, that is, those who embrace a spiritual worldview and those who embrace a materialist worldview. Having arrived on this planet, we look around and begin to formulate our worldview. According to Freud, we then make one of two basic assumptions: we view the universe as an accident and our existence as a matter of chance, or we assume some Intelligence beyond the universe and conclude that our existence has purpose in light of that Intelligence. Both worldviews begin with assumptions based on presuppositions that require considerable faith.

Freud's Worldview

As Freud described his worldview, we observe that he himself was not immune from making assertions based on philosophical assumptions rather than on research. For example, he began with the assumption that both the universe and life on this planet are a matter of chance. As Thomas Kuhn (1996) pointed out in his well-known book on scientific revolutions, a scientist's worldview influences not only what he investigates but how he perceives what he investigates. Kuhn wrote that two scientists with different views of the "order of nature...see different things when they look from the same point in the same direction.... they see different things and they see them in different relations to each other" (Kuhn 1996, p. 114). And we might add that they tend to see and to accept those data that conform to or make sense in light of that worldview.

Freud's assumptions led him to embrace a worldview that was strongly materialistic and dogmatically atheistic, a view that fueled his intense, lifelong attack on the spiritual worldview. The letters he wrote as an adolescent demonstrate that his worldview stemmed not from his clinical observations but preceded and influenced those observations.

When he was 18 years old, Freud wrote a letter to his college friend Edward Silberstein, the contents of which make it clear that he had already established his worldview. In that letter, Freud referred to himself as "a godless medical man." For a time, however, under the influence of a brilliant and devout professor of philosophy, Franz Brentano, Freud wavered. Freud wrote Silberstein that he was considering the "choice between theism and materialism" (Freud 1875/1991, p. 104). But this openness to a nonmaterialist worldview was only temporary. Throughout his life Freud referred to himself as an unbeliever. One year before his death, Freud wrote, "Neither in my private life nor in my writings have I ever made a secret of being an out-and-out unbeliever" (Freud 1938/1992, p. 453). In a letter to Oskar Pfister, the Swiss psychoanalyst and pastor, Freud asks, "Quite by the way, why did none of the devout create psychoanalysis? Why did one have to wait for a completely godless Jew?" (Freud 1918/1963, p. 63).

Many have wondered why Freud called himself an atheist and not an agnostic. Because a negative is impossible to prove, the position of atheism, which holds that God does not exist, is untenable on strictly logical grounds. During one of several visits to Hampstead, England, I asked Anna Freud why her father professed atheism rather than agnosticism. She answered by asking what the real difference was—and then explained that he believed religion was childishness and hoped that people would outgrow it. I asked about Einstein who Freud knew and respected and who professed a belief in God. She answered, "Yes, he did. But Einstein was also really very childlike." During the nineteenth century many scientists declared themselves atheists, which may explain Freud's comfort with atheism.

Much of Freud's writing during the last three decades of his life defined and defended this worldview. If we look in the general subject index of the standard edition of his complete works, we find many entries under the heading of "weltanschauung," many more than under what we would consider more popular psychoanalytic terms (Freud 1962). In his autobiography, Freud recalled "my early familiarity with the Bible story (at a time almost before I had learnt the art of reading) had, as I recognized much later, an enduring effect upon the direction of my interest" (Freud 1925/1962, p. 8). Then, in a postscript, Freud explained, "My interest after making a lifelong detour through the natural sciences, medicine and psychotherapy returned to the cultural problems which fascinated me long before, when I was a youth scarcely old enough for thinking" (Freud 1925/1962, p. 72).

Freud achieved his wish for cultural significance. In the seventeenth century, people turned to the discoveries of astronomy to demonstrate what they considered the irreconcilable conflict between science and faith; in the eighteenth century, to Newtonian physics; in the nineteenth century, to biology and Darwin; and in the twentieth century to Freud. Many scholars refer to the twentieth century as the century of Freud. Modern science tends to view faith as a psychological crutch, useful and perhaps necessary for the uneducated masses but out of the question as a viable modus operandi for the educated. One often hears in our universities that Freud proved God to be nothing but a figment of the mind. In addition, scholars have held the writings of Freud responsible in part for the secularization of our culture, for changing it from one in which the key values were primarily spiritual to one in which they are primarily material. Psychiatry continues to be considered by many as hostile to spiritual values.

Developmental Influences on Freud's Worldview

What influenced Freud to assert his militant materialistic worldview? Several influences—both external and internal—appear to have determined this view (Nicholi 2002).

One external influence was the cultural climate of the nineteenth century—a time when open warfare existed between science and religion. Freud spent the first half of his life in the last half of the nineteenth century. European culture at that time seethed with feelings of anticlericalism and contempt for all religious authority. A great deal of antireligious sentiment reflected reaction against the political powers of the Catholic Church. Most scientists clustered in one camp. Many of those admired by Freud embraced scientific positivism—the conviction that no truth existed outside of that derived from the laboratory. Many embraced atheism enthusiastically. Freud, who desperately wanted his new psychology to be accepted as science, had a vested interest in siding clearly with the scientists (Gay 1987, pp. 50–53).

The writings of Ludwig Feuerbach (1841/1989) provided another external influence. No individual influenced Freud more in the establishment of his atheism than this German philosopher. His writings formed the basis of the atheism not only of Marx and Engels but also of the young Freud. As a university student, Freud wrote a friend that, "among all philosophers I worship and admire (Feuerbach) the most" (Gay 1987, p. 53). Freud appears to have adopted the ideas of Feuerbach on religion in toto. Feuerbach wrote that God is a projection of man's inner needs and wishes and is therefore an illusion. (As so often happened in Freud's writings, Freud forgot to give Feuerbach credit for these ideas.)

One of the most significant inner determinants of Freud's atheism was his difficulty reconciling human suffering with a beneficent, omnipotent Creator. Freud himself suffered considerably, both *emotionally*, as a Jew growing up in an intensely Catholic society, and *physically*, with an intractable cancer of the palate that required many operations. He wrote repeatedly about the problem of reconciling human suffering with the existence of a beneficent God, which philosophers refer to as *theodicy*. For example, in a 1928 letter to Oskar Pfister, Freud lost his composure and became discourteous. He wrote, "And finally—let me be impolite for once—how the devil do you reconcile all that we experience and have come to expect in this world with your assumption of a moral world order?" (Freud 1928/1963, p. 123). In "The Question of a Weltanschauung," he wrote, "It seems not to be the case that there is a Power in the universe which watches over the well being of individuals with parental care and brings all their affairs to a happy ending.... Earthquakes, tidal waves, conflagrations make no distinction between the virtuous and pious and the scoundrel or unbeliever.... Obscure, unfeeling and unloving powers determine man's fate. The system of rewards and punishments which religion describes to the government of the universe seems not to exist" (Freud 1933/1962, p. 167).

However, the *primary* unconscious determinant of Freud's atheism may have been his intense unresolved ambivalence toward his father, Jacob Freud. His relationship with his father was a most unusual and complicated one. There is much evidence that this unresolved ambivalence formed the basis for Freud's hostile, persistent, emotionally charged attack on religion—Judaism as well as Christianity—as well as for his scientific contributions. For example, his oedipal theory formed the core of all his scientific contributions.

Freud's father Jacob was already a grandfather when he married Freud's mother, who was some 20 years younger. Thus, Freud was closer to his mother's age than was his father. Freud therefore was an uncle as soon as he was born. Freud's father died when Freud was about 40 years old. At that time Freud, through his own analysis, discovered within himself the passion for his young mother and the love and hatred for his father. On these feelings he based his idea of the Oedipus complex—what Ernest Jones, his official biographer, called "the greatest of all his original discoveries" (Jones 1957) and what Freud immodestly referred to as "among the precious new acquisitions of mankind" (Freud 1938/1962, p. 193). The evidence that this ambivalence was unresolved is substantial. Freud never had intercourse with his wife after his father's death. He described the death as "the most significant event" in his life and one that "revolutionized my soul." In one case history, Freud wrote that the patient, after his father's death, "denied himself all enjoyment of women out of a tender sense of guilt" (Freud 1922/1962, p. 228). Is it possible Freud himself had this same sense of guilt?

Freud associated his father with religious faith. Jacob Freud was educated as an Orthodox Jew. In 1891, he gave Freud for his 35th birthday a Bible with the following inscription in Hebrew:

> My dear son, It was in the seventh year of your life that the spirit of God began to move you to learning.... the spirit of God speaketh to you: 'Read in my book; there will be opened to you the sources of knowledge of the intellect...Thou has seen in this book the vision of the Almighty, Thou...has tried to fly high on the wings of the Holy Spirit. (Jones 1957, p. 19)

There can be no doubt Freud associated the spiritual worldview with his father.

Freud wrote about the intense negative feelings he harbored toward his father. Freud's father suffered financial reverses, and, with seven children to provide for, he had difficulty supporting Freud through his medical education. Freud saw his father as a failure. He recalled being bitterly disappointed as a little boy when his father refused to defend himself after being called a Jew by some anti-Semitic bullies and being pushed off the sidewalk (Jones 1957, p. 22). It seems likely that this unresolved ambivalence toward his father, the first authority in his life, influenced Freud's attitude toward all authority, including what he considered the Ultimate Authority. In a letter written in 1886 when he was 30 years old, Freud noted, "I always console myself with the thought that those subordinate to me or on the same level have never found me disagreeable, only those above me or who are in some other respect my superiors... I was always in vehement opposition to my teachers" (Jones 1957, p. 197).

Freud's Worldview and Clinical Work

Did Freud's atheism—his antispiritual worldview—influence his clinical observations?

Freud noticed from work with neurotic patients that unconscious attitudes toward authority figures—one's parents and especially one's father—may have a marked influence on one's conscious attitudes toward God. Freud wrote, "Let us transport ourselves into the mental life of a child—the mother who satisfies the child's hunger becomes the first love-object and certainly also the first protection against all the undefined dangers which threaten it in the external world—its first protection against anxiety, we may say. In this function [of protection], the mother is soon replaced by the stronger father who retains that position for the rest of childhood. But the child's attitude to its father is coloured by a *peculiar ambivalence*. The father constitutes a danger for the child, perhaps because of its earlier relation to its mother. Thus, it fears him no less than it longs for him and admires him" (Freud 1927/1962, pp. 23–24).

Freud observed that this yearning for an all-powerful father formed the basis for the adult's attitude toward God. Freud concluded that belief in God is an expression of powerful wishes and inner conflicts—a way of dealing with feelings of helplessness and with a strong wish for parental protection, especially that of the father. He noticed in some of his neurotic patients that when the authority of the father declined, the faith of these patients vanished.

Freud's observations can be verified clinically. Many who profess a faith have as the sole basis of that faith an unresolved, unconscious, or "neurotic" conflict. Their religious life has all of the manifestations of what we consider psychopathology. Psychodynamic psychiatry considers behavior pathological by the degree to which it is controlled by unconscious factors. The unconscious influences all behavior, but if it dominates behavior, that behavior manifests certain characteristics. Some of these characteristics are rigidity; stereotyped, repetitive, unalterable, and insatiable patterns; and inability to learn through experience or to be influenced by reason. Often, neurotic behavior tends to bring about what the person consciously wants most to avoid.

Patients whose spiritual convictions are based solely on neurotic need usually show two patterns of behavior. First, their behavior is grossly inconsistent with what they profess. Perhaps we have here a psychological explanation for the many ungodly acts throughout history that have been performed in the name of God—even acts of terrorism. Second, when the neurotic conflict of these patients has been resolved—in therapy or by other means—their faith often disappears.

Freud accurately observed many of the unconscious determinants of the faith of some of his neurotic patients and their tendency to displace childhood feelings from parental figures onto their concept of God. But his own bias against the spiritual worldview led him to draw several erroneous conclusions. Because Freud saw the element of wish fulfillment in the concept of God, he concluded that "God is psychologically nothing other than an exalted Father" (Freud 1913/1962). However, wishing for something has no real bearing on whether it exists. For example, the fact that most discoveries in medicine were wished for long before they were discovered does not make them less real.

Second, Freud, for his own reasons, failed to observe what he himself called "the deeper qualities" of faith, faith that was *not* neurotically determined, faith that Pfister, Freud's longtime friend, referred to as healthy and nonpathological. Freud insisted on exploring only what he called "the common man's religion," a distortion of biblical faith, and he explored this phenomenon only in neurotic patients. Third, he generalized from the beliefs of these few neurotic believers to all religious faith—even though he knew people such as Pfister, whom he admired immensely and whose faith he did not consider neurotic. Fourth, Freud's conclusion that all men wished for an omnipotent father contradicted what he considered the most important of his scientific discoveries. He failed to realize—or else ignored—that the negative part of ambivalent oedipal feelings may lead to neurotic antireligious convictions. Knowledge of the Oedipus complex leads one to expect that the unconscious wish that the all-powerful father *not* exist would be as strong, if not stronger than the wish that he *did* exist. Clinical evidence bears out this expectation in that the unbelief of some patients appears to be based on a strong unconscious (sometimes conscious) wish that God *not* exist. These examples illustrate how a clinician's worldview can lead to selective inattention and influence what he or she perceives and how he or she interprets what is perceived.

Freud's preoccupation with worldviews is clear. His collected works contain more than 150 references to God and more than 50 references to Jesus Christ. Freud's attempt to work out his own worldview and establish a philosophy of life caused him to focus his writings on issues that preoccupy the human spirit. These issues included an exploration of meaning and purpose, the universal search for happiness and for the reasons unhappiness prevails, the problem of pain and human suffering, the sources of morality and ethics, the existence of an Intelligence behind the universe, and the problem of human destiny, including what Freud called "the painful riddle of death." These themes, even more than his literary style and his scientific contributions, gave Freud's writings universal appeal and enduring influence.

One wonders whether Freud's interest ever entered the consulting room in the ways that this volume explores. Nevertheless, there are a few lessons we can learn from Freud's example that may serve as a point of departure for the chapters to come.

1. Freud's life calls attention to the importance of worldview. His intense attack on the spiritual worldview presents but one example of his recognition of this importance. Freud's writings illustrate the power of worldview in influencing both our approach to patients and our interpretation of scientific data.

2. Freud's materialistic worldview did not stem from his clinical observations and scientific discoveries but from cultural influences, such as the philosophical climate of his day, and from his early life experiences. His

worldview was formed long before he began his scientific work, and considerable evidence exists that his worldview strongly influenced what he observed and what he failed to observe clinically. Everyone possesses a worldview, a philosophy of life. Whether we realize it or not, that worldview determines in large measure who we are and how we function as investigators and clinicians. An awareness of our worldview may help us understand not only the ways in which we perceive clinically but also our biases, the tendencies that can impair our clinical effectiveness.

3. No clinician, regardless of clinical skills, can know the patient without exploring that patient's weltanschauung. The patient's worldview gives the clinician insight into the patient's self-image, relationships, values, and identity, as well as how he or she confronts illness, suffering, and death. A clinician's understanding of the patient's worldview, as well as the clinician's insight into his or her own worldview, provides the key to establishing the most salubrious doctor–patient relationship.

References

Feuerbach L: The Essence of Christianity (1841). Translated by George Eliot. Amherst, NY, Prometheus Books, 1989

Freud S: Letter to Eduard Silberstein (1875), in The Letters of Sigmund Freud to Eduard Silberstein 1871–1881. Edited by Boehlich W. Translated by Pomerans AJ. Cambridge, MA, Belknap Press of Harvard University Press, 1991

Freud S: Totem and taboo (1913), in The Standard Edition of the Complete Psychological Works of Sigmund Freud, Vol 13. Translated and edited by Strachey J. London, Hogarth Press, 1962, pp 1–161

Freud S: Letter to Oskar Pfister (1918), in Psychoanalysis and Faith: The Letters of Sigmund Freud and Oskar Pfister. Edited by Meng H, Freud EL. New York, Basic Books, 1963

Freud S: Some neurotic mechanisms in jealousy, paranoia and homosexuality (1922) in The Standard Edition of the Complete Psychological Works of Sigmund Freud, Vol 18. Translated and edited by Strachey J. London, Hogarth Press, 1962, pp 221–232

Freud S: An autobiographical study (1925), in The Standard Edition of the Complete Psychological Works of Sigmund Freud, Vol 20. Translated and edited by Strachey J. London, Hogarth Press, 1962, pp 1–71

Freud S: Future of an illusion (1927), in The Standard Edition of the Complete Psychological Works of Sigmund Freud, Vol 21. Translated and edited by Strachey J. London, Hogarth Press, 1962, pp 5–56

Freud S: Letter to Oskar Pfister (1928), in Psychoanalysis and Faith: The Letters of Sigmund Freud and Oskar Pfister. Edited by Meng H, Freud EL. New York, Basic Books, 1963, p 123

Freud S: The question of a weltanschauung (1933), in The Standard Edition of the Complete Psychological Works of Sigmund Freud, Vol 22. Translated and edited by Strachey J. London, Hogarth Press, 1962, pp 158–182

Freud S: Letter of Sigmund Freud (1938), in Letters of Sigmund Freud, 1873–1939. Edited by Freud EL. Translated by Stein T, Stein J. New York, Dover Publications, 1992

Freud S: An outline of psycho-analysis (1938), in The Standard Edition of the Complete Psychological Works of Sigmund Freud, Vol 23. Translated and edited by Strachey J. London, Hogarth Press, 1962, pp 144–207

Freud S: Indexes and bibliographies (1962), in The Standard Edition of the Complete Psychological Works of Sigmund Freud, Vol 24. Translated and edited by Strachey J. London, Hogarth Press, 1962, pp 3–468

Gay P: A Godless Jew: Freud, Atheism, and the Making of Psychoanalysis. New Haven, CT, Yale University Press, 1987

Jones E: The Life and Work of Sigmund Freud, Vol 1: The Formative Years and the Great Discoveries (1856–1900). New York, Basic Books, 1957

Kuhn TS: The Structure of Scientific Revolutions, 3rd Edition. Chicago, IL, University of Chicago Press, 1996

Nicholi AM: The Question of God: CS Lewis and Sigmund Freud Debate God, Love, Sex, and the Meaning of Life. New York, Free Press, 2002

PART II

Clinical Foundations

CHAPTER 2

Worldview in Psychiatric Assessment

Allan M. Josephson, M.D.
Irving S. Wiesner, M.D.

Historically, psychiatry and psychology adopted an approach that was consistent with the development of science. This approach dictated that only phenomena that could be reliably observed, measured, or described were proper subjects of the scientific endeavor. The clinical assessment of other phenomena was not seen as important, and, as a result, religion and spirituality were relegated to the sidelines. Freud (1913/1962) then introduced the concept that religion was immature (wish fulfillment) and further discouraged clinicians from taking it seriously. This attitude did not, however, remove religion and spirituality from importance in patients' lives. Psychiatry's understanding of religion as a risk factor for some types of psychopathology has since been balanced by evidence that religious factors may protect certain individuals from psychological symptoms (Josephson et al. 2000; Koenig 1998; Larson et al. 1992).

Religious and spiritual issues are inextricably woven into patients' lives and may influence their disorders as well. Although the clinical influence of these issues varies from patient to patient, the assessment of the patient's worldview—of his or her religious, spiritual, or philosophical outlook on life—is relevant to both diagnostic formulation and treatment planning, which are discussed in Chapters 3 and 4, "Worldview in Diagnosis and Case Formulation" and "Therapeutic Implications of Worldview," respectively. This chapter will review key reasons for conducting a spiritual, religious, or philosophical assessment and examine some factors that influence the process of gathering this information, the fundamental types of data obtained in the assessment, and some situations in which a more in-depth assessment of worldview may be appropriate. These topics have been addressed by other authors (Chirban 2001; Gorsuch and Miller 1999; Richards and Bergin 1997; Wiesner 1996), and the reader is referred to the earlier works for further study. Whether the assessment is done briefly or in depth, a basic understanding of the patient's worldview is a vital component of any psychiatric evaluation and should be part of the practice of all well-trained psychiatrists (American Medical Association 2002).

One's worldview, or philosophical outlook on life, may or may not be religiously based, but it inevitably includes assumptions about the larger context of human existence (see Chapter 1, "Introduction: Definition and Significance of a Worldview"). Since most patients think about their relationship to this context in spiritual terms, the remainder of this chapter refers, for simplicity, to the religious or spiritual assessment. (Atheists and agnostics also have attitudes toward religion and spirituality that may be clinically relevant.) The terms religion and spirituality are often used synonymously but are actually separate, yet related, aspects of life experience. As the term is generally used, *spirituality* refers to one's connection to realities larger than oneself or larger than the material universe. It is an umbrella concept under which the specific category of *religion* is subsumed. The tendency to believe that there is more to existence than the material—that life has a spiritual element—is codified in various religions through beliefs and related historical events, or tenets, that are usually documented in written form (scriptures). Religions formalize what the spiritual individual experiences. Religious expressions include cognitive elements (beliefs and theology) and behavioral elements, such as ritual and spiritual experience (e.g., prayers and religious services). Religious expressions are typically codified and as such are inevitably tied to specific traditions.

Reasons for Conducting a Religious or Spiritual Assessment

There are several reasons why clinicians should assess the patient's religious and spiritual life:

1. Religion and spirituality may contribute to the risk of developing a clinical problem, or they may serve as protective factors. The refusal of a rigid, religious family to allow an adolescent to question religious dogma can become a focus of the adolescent's oppositional behavior; one could

imagine that the family's reaction to the adolescent's drug use would have a similar effect. On the other hand, a religious family that has provided a structured, nurturing environment with clear explication of moral codes may protect an adolescent from substance abuse (Miller et al. 2000). Careful assessment is necessary to determine whether religion is promoting health or disorder, so that this information can be appropriately integrated into the treatment plan.

2. Religious and spiritual assessment can improve the treatment alliance. All patients desire to be understood and are more likely to follow the recommendations of a clinician whom they perceive to understand them empathically. By the same token, the patient with strong religious or spiritual inclinations may feel rebuffed if a clinician either actively or passively avoids asking about issues that the patient considers so important. This concern may be less central if the patient is irreligious or has a secular outlook, but if a religious or spiritual tradition has been important to the patient or the patient's family, an assessment of this area adds legitimacy to the clinical encounter and likely heightens the patient's confidence in the clinician. When the clinician and patient share a particular worldview or spiritual tradition, this mutual background may facilitate a deeper understanding of the patient's clinical problems and their context.

3. Religious and spiritual assessment can reveal resources within a patient's religious beliefs or religious community that could facilitate treatment. At times, an assessment can lead to the clinician's establishing a natural collaboration with clergy or others in the patient's faith community. This collaboration can tap sources of support for the patient and may serve as a type of consultation for the clinician by deepening his or her understanding of the religious beliefs and spiritual traditions of the patient.

4. The patient's problem may present within a religious or spiritual context, which needs to be explored. The following case vignette illustrates this clinical situation:

> A 29-year-old man presented with a loss of sleep and concentration shortly after his 18-year-old brother died of leukemia. The patient previously had a strong religious background and yet began to wonder whether God exists. These doubts in turn caused him significant anxiety.

5. The clinical situation may suggest that existential or moral issues are prominent. Examples include clinical syndromes that may arise when an individual faces a life-threatening illness in him- or herself or in a family member or faces a dilemma with moral dimensions, such as the decision to divorce.

6. Patients may cite religious reasons for their difficulty in accepting psychotherapy, pharmacotherapy, or medical therapies. An in-depth reli-

gious and spiritual history that distinguishes religious from other forms of resistance can foster compliance with treatment.

7. Raising children typically involves inculcating values and explicating moral codes. These parental actions help children develop internalized control over impulses and foster development. Managing certain developmental needs of children can be problematic for many parents, particularly when the children are experiencing the onset of adolescent sexuality. As many parental responses have a basis in a religious or spiritual tradition, an assessment of these factors is usually indicated.

General Considerations Regarding the Interview

The religious and spiritual assessment fits within the psychiatric interview, the cornerstone of the diagnostic process. Before focusing on the content of the assessment, it is important to note that the manner in which one conducts a religious and spiritual assessment may be as important as the facts that are obtained.

Interviewing involves gathering facts and listening to the patient's narrative, while also balancing the science of description with the clinical art of following the patient. Patients often express spiritual experiences through metaphor and story. Griffith and Griffith (2002) described the manner in which the clinician's openness in following the patient's story, in contrast to "peppering" the patient with questions, often leads to an elaboration of religious and spiritual material. Through this elaboration, experiences and beliefs are intermingled as the patient describes religious and spiritual phenomena. Thus, the spiritual interview is consistent with effective psychodynamic interviewing. Based on their practice, Griffith and Griffith argued that patients more often desire a spiritual experience than a religious explanation. As they put it, "God objectifies the relatedness of spirituality" (Griffith and Griffith 2002, p. 17). In fact, patients often emphasize both. In the process of the religious and spiritual assessment, the clinician listens for the patient's *beliefs* about God and his or her spiritual *experience* of the transcendent.

Griffith and Griffith referred to Kahle's unpublished research on therapists' behavior in which most of the therapists who were surveyed said that they would follow religious questioning if the patient initiated the topic of faith (Griffith and Griffith 2002, p. 31). However, a much smaller number of therapists said they would ask questions about God and spirituality on their own initiative. When asked about factors that influenced their decision of whether to ask about spirituality, the surveyed therapists cited their professional education as a factor that discouraged spiritual questions and the obvious interest of the patients themselves as a factor that encouraged this questioning. It appears many clinicians proceed with this type of interview with some degree of reticence. The clinician should counteract this natural tendency with attention to material that may suggest a spiritual or religious interest, including developmental and psychodynamic factors. The goal is to understand the role of spiritual factors in any formulation (see Chapter 3, "Worldview in Diagnosis and Case Formulation"). During the interview, the clinician should be prepared to respond to questions the patient may ask about the clinician's own religious or spiritual background. The therapeutic boundary issues implicit in this point will be covered in Chapter 4, "Therapeutic Implications of Worldview."

The American Psychiatric Association recommends that psychiatrists should not only maintain respect for their patient's beliefs but consider that "it is useful for clinicians to obtain information on the religious or ideological orientation and beliefs of their patients so that they may properly attend to them in the course of treatment" (American Psychiatric Association 1990, p. 542). One of the tenets of this book is that the patient's worldview and the physician's worldview interact in important ways. Even though effective interviewing may seem technically neutral, the manner in which the interview is conducted is greatly influenced by the clinician's worldview. For example, distinguishing between psychopathology and spiritual or religious beliefs is an objective determination, yet one that is powerfully, if subtly, influenced by the clinician's own belief system.

The APA guidelines also encourage clinicians to use empathic responses to the patient's particular beliefs and to respect their value and meaning to the patient. However, the religious and spiritual assessment of the patient has the potential for strong countertransference elements that can evoke uncomfortable feelings for therapists. These feelings can lead to various interviewing problems. Some therapists may ignore religious material because of awkwardness or ignorance, while others who have negative feelings about religious material may be unable to facilitate an effective discussion of these issues. On the other hand, clinicians who have a positive view of spirituality and religion may have other problems. They may not confront the patient's religiously based pathology, because they may feel too closely aligned with the patient's faith position. Awareness that such factors may influence the assessment will improve a clinician's understanding of how his or her worldview is likely to affect the clinical encounter.

Referral patterns may influence whether a religious and spiritual assessment takes place and, if it takes place, how extensive it is. Most patients have some knowledge of the type of psychiatric or mental health care facilities in their communities, and many seek out particular clinics because of their reputation for excellent management of specific disorders. Some explicitly religious mental health clinics exist (for example, those in religious institutions), but for the most part, individuals who are seeking care do not know the religious or spiritual orientation of a given practitioner or clinic. At the same time, clergy in many religious and spiritual traditions have become increasingly sensitive to and knowledgeable about mental health interventions, and they may refer individuals to clinicians whom they know are open to religious and spiritual issues and supportive of religious health (Larson et al. 1988).

The initial clinical setting will also influence the type of religious and spiritual assessment. An evaluation of an acutely psychotic patient in an emergency setting will focus on differential diagnosis and a safe, immediate intervention. Psychotic religious content may be meaningful, but the clinician will need to wait until the patient is more stable before conducting a religious and spiritual assessment.

Consultation on the medical floor of a general hospital may require a religious and spiritual assessment if a patient's refusal of a procedure is based on religious belief, as it may be if the patient is a Jehovah's Witness. A consultation to a dying patient on an oncology unit may require an understanding of the patient's spiritual tradition in order to help the patient cope with existential questions arising in the midst of life-threatening illness. An outpatient psychiatric evaluation in a private clinic may only briefly address spiritual issues, but the clinician may, through a deepening understanding of the patient's beliefs, focus more on spiritual or religious issues as psychotherapy proceeds.

Screening Versus Complete Assessment

In most cases, the religious and spiritual assessment is not a primary emphasis of the psychiatric interview. Basic spiritual or religious elements should be addressed with all patients in a routine screening that is similar to the brief screening for vegetative signs of depression and vocational or educational history. Patients typically expect such a review of life factors. The clinician must also be attuned to indications that religion and spirituality are important to the patient. Such indications may include the nature of the patient's clothing or the type of reading material the patient has brought with him or her. The importance of religion and spirituality may become evident when the patient asks about the clinician's religious background or moral views regarding specific behaviors.

Some clinicians augment the interview with screening instruments. Richards and Bergin (1997) have suggested questions related to the patient's current religious affiliation, developmental history, overall worldview, and specific religious or current concerns. However, they noted that research measures in the area of religion have not been standardized for use in clinical situations. In addition, most self-report measures for religious and spiritual assessment have been developed within the framework of Christian theology and are not relevant for non-Christian patients.

Koenig and Pritchett (1998) reported on use of a brief screen with the acronym FICA to help structure such questions:

F—Is religious *faith* an important part of your day-to-day life? This question could be followed by associated questions about formal religious identity and level of spirituality.

I—How has faith *influenced* your life, past and present? This question may uncover important spiritual experiences.

C—Are you currently a part of a religious or spiritual *community*? This question helps clarify the role a spiritual community might play in treatment interventions.

A—What are the spiritual needs that you would like me to *address*? This question allows the clinician to identify spiritual areas that may be part of a treatment plan.

In response to screening questions, patients may give answers that indicate no further need to proceed with questioning about spiritual or religious matters. This situation is analogous to a patient's providing negative responses to screening questions about educational or vocational history or to a review of physical systems. However, such responses do not mean that religion or spirituality is not important or will not resurface in later clinical contacts. In some instances, in the initial assessment, the patient may be reticent to share religious beliefs or spiritual experiences, similar to a patient's withholding of sensitive material about sexual matters. The clinician should recognize that screening and initial assessments may be cursory and that only later, in the deepening of a psychotherapeutic treatment, may important religious and spiritual material emerge.

In the initial screening, some patients give responses that indicate a need for further, in-depth evaluation of spiritual or religious issues. Richards and Bergin (1997) called this in-depth assessment a "Level Two" evaluation, in contrast to a "Level One" screening examination. An in-depth religious and spiritual assessment includes consideration of both process and content.

Process of the In-Depth Interview

Following the patient by means of sensitive yet probing questions, the interviewer tries to uncover spiritual material through a naturally unfolding process, as illustrated in the following account:

A 31-year-old single pregnant woman presented with the chief complaint that "I'm stressed out…I'm pregnant, and I lost my job." In the course of providing a full family history, she reported that her 21-year-old sister had died of lymphoma 10 years earlier and that she had required psychiatric treatment at that time, albeit briefly. Later in the evaluation, after a systematic review of her medical and educational history, she was asked about her religious faith. She responded that she had none. For further clarification, she was then asked whether she had been raised in a particular faith and responded, "Methodist." "So religion is not an important part of your life?" she was asked. Her reply revealed potential avenues of further inquiry: "Not an important part of my life since my sister died…. It's not that I don't believe in God, I just stopped going to church." Going a step further, the clinician asked what she believed happens after death. "I believe we go to heaven," she said. "Everyone?" she was asked. "I don't know if I believe in hell," she replied, "I think we are all in it here sometimes."

This interviewer probed beyond the point at which some interviewers may have ceased questioning. At the same time, the probing was sensitive and empathic and ultimately revealed existential material related to the patient's current pervasive hopelessness.

Sometimes patients ask questions about issues with moral and religious overtones.

A 41-year-old mother was discussing the behavior problems of her 15-year-old son with a child and adolescent psychiatrist. In sharing information about her son's school performance and behavior, she related that recently her female partner had moved in to live with her and her son. She wondered whether this change had affected his academic performance and then blurted out, "Do you think homosexuality is wrong?" In asking questions about the therapist's personal views, the mother revealed her own intense interest in the views of others on this subject.

In such instances, process-oriented interviews can yield valuable material, sometimes through the use of projective questions. For example, a patient who identifies himself as being thoroughly familiar with the Old Testament could be asked to name the most interesting personality he finds in the scriptures. If he chooses David, the Old Testament shepherd boy who later became the king of Israel, he may explain his choice by saying that "David was interesting because he was such a little guy and was able to kill that big giant" or that David is to be admired "because he committed adultery and murder and got away with it." Or finally, perhaps David may be interesting because he was known as "a man after God's own heart." Such projective questioning has value in revealing general psychodynamic issues as well as spiritual material (Draper et al. 1965). In the process-oriented interview, most patients give clues that they are open to further questions.

When religious issues are directly associated with presenting symptoms, there is less need to probe in the interview. In those situations, the exploration of religious issues is simply part of a thorough review of the presenting complaint.

For example, a 38-year-old woman presented with guilt associated with a depressive disorder and reported that the syndrome developed after she had an abortion. She described the guilt as based, in large part, on her religious beliefs. When the patient presents such issues as linked to psychiatric symptoms, the clinician must assess the areas of spirituality and religion. It is possible that religious and spiritual data are not directly relevant to a case formulation, but this possibility can be evaluated only after all the relevant information has been gathered. The clinician may err in two directions: by overly exploring the patient's religious and spiritual background or by ignoring this area altogether.

Content of the In-Depth Interview: Clinical Categories

When the patient does not report that religious issues are associated with the presenting complaint, the clinician may still have an index of suspicion that religious belief or spiritual practice has a role in the patient's psychopathology and should be considered in treatment planning. This sense is particularly useful to pursue when there are clinically meaningful data in the following areas or categories.

Spiritual Manifestations of Psychiatric Disorder

Specific psychiatric disorders, demonstrated to have strong biological loading, may have apparent religious components. These elements include religious obsessions in obsessive-compulsive disorder, feelings of being influenced by divine powers in schizophrenia, and religious delusions of grandiosity in mania. In these instances, the clinician gathers the apparent religious data along with the data on other symptoms.

Religious Factors That Influence Clinical Problems

Religious factors may predispose the patient to the development of clinical problems or may perpetuate existing clinical problems.

> A 42-year-old man with a persistent pattern of job loss was terminated from employment. His past substance abuse problem recurred, and he became increasingly anxious and full of rage at his employer. A review of his spiritual history revealed that he was the son of a minister, and his developmental years were spent in a rigid family that did not tolerate religious questioning.

He became an atheist in his young adult life and has struggled in situations that require his acceptance of authority.

Existential Issues Related to Death, Suffering, and Interpersonal Loss

Ironically, personal transformation can sometimes result when individuals are forced to question the meaning of their lives, even when this questioning can be so intense that it mimics a psychiatric condition. For example, a successful lawyer pursued a political career and achieved political success beyond his expectations. After he had achieved what he perceived to be the pinnacle of his career, he seriously questioned his motives and wondered about the origins of his paradoxical despondency. He subsequently had a religious conversion experience and devoted the next phase of his life to self-sacrificial community service.

Moral Failings Associated With Psychiatric Symptoms

Guilt associated with perceived moral failings may be appropriate, as in the case of a patient whose extramarital affair precipitates a divorce that hurts his or her children. This realistic guilt is contrasted with the inappropriate guilt of the individual who has difficulty enjoying sexuality due to a harsh, restrictive religious upbringing.

Religious or Spiritual Problems

Religious or spiritual problems can be a legitimate focus of clinical attention apart from any psychiatric syndrome. For example, clinical attention may be sought by individuals who experience a loss of faith or who question their faith, have problems associated with conversion to a new faith, or question their spiritual values (American Psychiatric Association 2000, p. 741).

Protective Functions of Religious or Spiritual Factors

Individuals may report that their faith or spiritual practice has helped reduce their symptoms or provided significant support. Even if the patient does not mention religion or spirituality as a source of support, the clinician should always inquire about the availability of a religious or spiritual community, which may be an asset in treatment planning.

A 36-year-old, twice married mother of a 5-year-old daughter presented for help with the child's disruptive behavior. It was clear to the assessing clinician that the mother had experienced a depressive disorder, had struggled with substance abuse, and was in an unsupportive marriage. When asked about her sources of support, she responded, "My depression never really got better until I began to worship God. The people at the church are great; they really care about me."

Content of the In-Depth Interview: Spiritual Categories

Exploration of clinically meaningful categories often reveals the need for questioning about specific spiritual areas. The clinical interviewer may encourage discussion of these areas by using the guide questions shown in Table 2–1 that are relevant to the patient's situation.

Developmental History

Since one component of family process is spiritual or religious experience, the gathering of information about spiritual development fits naturally into a review of the family's developmental experience (Coles 1990). Was spirituality or religion a part of family life, or were there mentors outside the family who had spiritual influence? It is important to get some sense of the patient's frequency of attending religious services during the developmental years and of whether religion or spirituality was a source of conflict between family members or with others outside the family. In the process of development, the patient may have experienced dramatic changes in spiritual or religious traditions either toward a tradition (a "conversion") or away from one. It is crucial to understand these transitions, as they often have profound significance for understanding a patient's current functioning. Assessment includes evaluation of the maturity of the patient's faith development (Fowler 1981) and of the patient's current sense of spiritual well-being, which is often closely tied to his or her sense of acceptance by a higher power.

Community

It is important to appreciate whether the patient is a member of a specific religious or spiritual community. Knowledge of the patients' current identification with a religious or spiritual community and of the practices of that community are helpful in understanding the individual's religious or spiritual network. Religious and spiritual communities can be a source of support in dealing with mental disorders, but conflicts within the community can be a source of stress for the patient. This potential source of distress should not be underestimated. The patient's religious or spiritual community may play a central role in his or her life, and any disparity between the community's standards and the patient's current behavior can be a source of significant stress. It is important to understand the community's view of mental disorders and whether the community has recently undergone any significant changes.

TABLE 2–1.	Interview guide for the in-depth spiritual and religious assessment

I. **Developmental history**

   1. Describe your first religious experience or belief.
   2. Do you have childhood religious memories?
   3. Describe your religious education or training.
   4. Describe your parents' religious or spiritual beliefs and practices.
   5. Did they behave in a manner consistent with their expressed beliefs?
   6. Are your beliefs similar to those of your parents? Do they differ? In what way?
   7. Were any other people important to your religious experiences? Who?
   8. Did you have any religious experiences you felt were traumatic?
   9. Did you have an experience where you changed your religious or spiritual views (e.g., a conversion)?
   10. Do you desire to develop spiritually? In what way?

II. **Community**

   1. Do you participate in church or synagogue life now?
   2. Have you changed churches (religions, synagogues) as an adult? Why?
   3. What is the most meaningful support you have received from a spiritual community?
   4. Do you try to get others to join your religious community?

III. **God**

   1. Do you believe in the existence of a God? What led you to this belief?
   2. Do you not believe in the existence of God? What led you to this belief?
   3. Describe God's characteristics.
   4. How does belief in God affect your personal experience?
   5. Is God a person to you, a force, or an idea?
   6. How do you experience God? Does God speak to you? Have you had special experiences with God?

IV. **Belief**

   1. What is your single most important religious belief?
   2. Which of your religious beliefs do you doubt the most?
   3. What religious beliefs do you doubt the least?
   4. Are you troubled by evil or suffering in the world? What causes it?
   5. For you, what is a life with purpose?

V. **Rituals and practices**

   1. What does prayer mean to you?
   2. If you pray, what do you pray for?
   3. How often do you pray? Do you pray alone or with others?
   4. Do you engage in other private religious practices, such as rituals or study of scriptures? How often?
   5. How often do you attend spiritual or religious services?

TABLE 2–1.	Interview guide for the in-depth spiritual and religious assessment *(continued)*

VI. Spiritual Experience
   1. Have you had experiences that you would describe as spiritual?
   2. Did these experiences change the direction of your life?
   3. Have you told others about these experiences?
   4. How important is spiritual experience to your daily life?

God

It is important for the clinician to inquire about the patient's spiritual or religious concept of God and the patient's view about what is of ultimate importance. Is God perceived as a "force" or a "person"? Is God loving, kind, and forgiving or wrathful, impersonal, and vindictive? A God image is the person's perception or mental representation of God, which is not necessarily what he or she has been taught about God. There are several reasons why an assessment should seek to understand how patients perceive God. One of the most important is that perceptions of God are often connected to perceptions of parents, significant others, and the self. Insight into the patient's image of God helps the clinician understand the patient's other internalized object relations (Rizzuto 1979).

Belief

It is possible to distinguish three major spiritual or religious traditions. Abramic traditions trace their history to Abraham and adhere to the doctrines of creation, fall, and redemption. This tradition includes Judaism, Christianity, and Islam. Yogic traditions, exemplified by Hinduism and Buddhism, believe in karma and rebirth (reincarnation). Devotees follow gurus in learning yoga and meditation. The naturalistic or materialistic position, while often not seen as a spiritual or religious tradition, nevertheless has a worldview. Individuals with this "tradition" believe that the universe has no purpose or reason and that truth can be known only through scientific means. Atheists, materialists, and many agnostics believe that rational thought is the highest form of human consciousness and, therefore, the arbiter of truth or falsehood.

Assessing belief is important since the "thought is the mother to the deed." In some religious or spiritual traditions, formal beliefs are emphasized over the individual's experience, but to avoid inquiring about beliefs for this reason would be an error. In addition to assessing formal religious belief and theological tenets, it is important to assess informal beliefs, such as a belief in parapsychology. Most religious traditions vary on a spectrum from liberal to fundamental, which increases the complexity of assessing this area.

At times, inquiring about a patient's beliefs and source of morality can reveal the basis for unexplained symptoms.

> A 17-year-old high school senior was referred for psychiatric evaluation after medical evaluation for headache and abdominal pain did not reveal any known organic cause. As part of routine history, she told the psychiatrist that she had been homeschooled after attending a parochial school much of her life. When the psychiatrist inquired about her family's faith background, she responded tersely, "Faith! Faith! That's my whole problem." This outburst was followed by a description of a rigid, authoritarian relationship with a priest who had insisted that all anger was sinful. Through the recognition of the validity of some of her anger and the behavioral necessity of expressing it, her symptoms began to resolve. She came to understand the relationship of her beliefs to her symptoms.

Any unusual symptom, such as guilt about sexual behavior, that appears to have a basis in specific beliefs should be explored to see what the patient believes to be the source of ultimate knowledge—for example, authority (often concretized through sacred scriptures), reason, or experience. Some specific and unique beliefs may require a religious interpreter.

Rituals and Practices

The commonest rituals and practices in most religious and spiritual traditions are prayer and meditation. The role such practices play in the patient's life—how, how often, and why they are undertaken—reveal character structure, dynamic conflicts, and sources of strength, as well as the extent of religious devotion. Extremely devout patients may have specific requirements of worship, fasting, and service that are part of their day-to-day life.

Spiritual Experiences

Finally, it may be important to explore the individual's spiritual experience. Many religious individuals emphasize either belief or experience to an extreme; those with healthy adaptations usually acknowledge the importance of both. Some spiritual experiences are so transcendent that they are described as life changing. Some experiences can be negative and traumatic, such as forced indoctrination or abuse by clergy.

Summary

Clinicians should gather basic data on spiritual and religious experience from all patients, as this information provides a background for comprehensive care. At the end of the religious or spiritual component of the psychiatric assessment, the clinician should have an opinion about the importance of religion and spirituality in the patient's life and about the relative health or pathology of the patient's beliefs and experiences in this area. The clinician should also know when it is clinically indicated to gather more detailed religious and spiritual information and how to do so. In addition, the clinician should be alert to the manner in which his or her own worldview influences the exploration of religious and spiritual issues and the importance they are given in diagnostic formulation.

References

American Medical Association: Program requirements for residency education in psychiatry, in Graduate Medical Education Directory, 2002–2003. Chicago, IL, American Medical Association, 2002, pp 309–317

American Psychiatric Association: Guidelines regarding possible conflict between psychiatrists' religious commitments and psychiatric practice. Am J Psychiatry 147:542, 1990

American Psychiatric Association: Diagnostic and Statistical Manual of Mental Disorders 4th Edition. Washington, DC, American Psychiatric Association, 1994

Chirban J: Assessing religious and spiritual concerns in psychotherapy, in Faith and Health: Perspectives on the Relationship Between Religious Faith and Health Outcomes. Edited by Plante TG, Sherman AC. New York, Guilford, 2001, pp 265–290

Coles R: The Spiritual Life of Children. Boston, MA, Houghton Mifflin, 1990

Draper E, Meyer GG, Parze Z, et al: On the diagnostic value of religious ideation. Arch Gen Psychiatry 13:202–207, 1965

Fowler JW: Stages of Faith. San Francisco, CA, Harper and Row, 1981

Freud S: Totem and taboo (1913), in the Standard Edition of the Complete Psychological Works of Sigmund Freud, Vol. 13. Translated and edited by Strachey J. London, Hogarth Press, 1962, pp 1–61

Gorsuch RL, Miller WR: Assessing spirituality, in Integrating Spirituality Into Treatment. Edited by Miller WR. Washington, DC, American Psychological Association, 1999, pp 147–164

Griffith JL, Griffith ME: Encountering the Sacred in Psychotherapy: How to Talk With People About Their Spiritual Lives. New York, Guilford, 2002

Josephson AM, Larson, DB, Juthani N: What's happening in psychiatry regarding spirituality. Psychiatr Ann 30:533–541, 2000

Koenig HG (ed): Handbook of Religion and Mental Health. San Diego, CA, Academic Press, 1998

Koenig HG, Pritchett J: Religion and psychotherapy, in Handbook of Religion and Mental Health. Edited by Koenig HG. San Diego, CA, Academic Press, 1998, pp 323–336

Larson DB, Hohmann AA, Kessler LG, et al: The couch and the cloth: the need for linkage. Hosp Community Psychiatry 39:1064–1069, 1988

Larson DB, Sherrill KA, Lyons JS, et al: Associations between dimensions of religious commitment and mental health reported in the American Journal of Psychiatry and Archives of General Psychiatry: 1978–1989. Am J Psychiatry 149:527–559, 1992

Miller L, Davies M, Greenwald S: Religiosity and substance use and abuse among adolescents in the National Comorbidity Survey. J Am Acad Child Adolesc Psychiatry 39:1190–1197, 2000

Richards PS, Bergin A: A Spiritual Strategy for Counseling and Psychotherapy. Washington, DC, American Psychological Association, 1997

Rizzuto AM: The Birth of the Living God: A Psychoanalytic Inquiry. Chicago, IL, University of Chicago Press, 1979

Wiesner IS: The clinical exploration of the patient's world view. Directions in Psychiatry 16:1–8, 1996

CHAPTER 3

Worldview in Diagnosis and Case Formulation

Allan M. Josephson, M.D.

John R. Peteet, M.D.

Once information has been gathered through the psychiatric interview, a clinician faces the task of bringing an often overwhelming amount of clinical material together into a meaningful narrative, which is the basis for comprehensive treatment. What information is essential to understanding the patient—for example, a rigid religious background that has apparently facilitated a patient's oppositional style and rush to atheism? What information is ancillary—for example, a patient's nominal Catholicism? How related are the patient's presenting clinical problems to his or her worldview? Are there spiritual and religious resources for healing? This chapter offers guidelines for using the information gathered during the clinical assessment (see Chapter 2, "Worldview in Psychiatric Assessment") to develop a diagnostic case formulation that can serve as a basis for appropriate and effective treatment (see Chapter 4, "Therapeutic Implications of Worldview"). The development of the formulation is a critical step in this process since it determines whether the clinician sees the patient's spirituality and beliefs as risk factors for psychopathology (requiring intervention directed toward change) or as protective or supportive of health (in need of facilitation).

Integrating Spirituality and Worldview Into a "Biopsychosociospiritual" Formulation

The word diagnosis comes from the Greek *dia*, meaning through, and *gnosis*, referring to knowledge. Diagnosis then is knowing through or knowing deeply. Descriptive DSM-IV-TR nomenclature offers an initial, categorizing approach, and the case formulation is an attempt at "knowing" a patient more deeply. The process of developing the formulation begins the minute a patient has clinical contact with the clinician and continues throughout therapy. Time is often necessary to facilitate a deeper understanding of the patient in sensitive areas such as sexuality and spirituality.

Engel (1977) coined the term "biopsychosocial" to assist physicians in the diagnostic process as they gathered all data relevant to the onset, maintenance, and perpetuation of a disorder. Initially applied in internal medicine, this idea has received particular attention in psychiatry because of its usefulness in helping clinicians avoid the reductionism inherent in attributing complex disorders to a single cause (Engel 1980). In this chapter, the term *case formulation* refers not simply to a psychodynamic hypothesis but to a comprehensive consideration of relevant etiologic and protective factors in a given patient's case. Since one of these factors is often the internalized psychological worldview of the patient, it seems appropriate to broaden Engel's term to include the spiritual, hence our reference to an even more cumbersome term, the *biopsychosociospiritual* formulation.

The soundly constructed biopsychosociospiritual case formulation has several characteristics. It balances consideration of biological, psychological, social, and spiritual factors in conceptualizing the etiology of a disorder. It is consistent with an organism-environment interactive process and consistent with available empirical data, which can be used as a guide to the development of the formulation (e.g., empirical evidence of the association between abuse and dissociative disorders). Finally, such a formulation is supported by clinical data. Speculative formulations that are not grounded in these ways reveal more about the biases of the clinician than about the patient.

Some clinicians may regard a patient's spiritual and religious experience as fitting more appropriately into the category of social factors, rather than deserving separate consideration. Admittedly, it is often difficult to determine which factor is primary—culture, ethnicity, or spirituality or religion.

A 14-year-old girl was treated for obsessive-compulsive disorder. Pharmacotherapy was somewhat ineffective, as it was undermined by a family constellation of overprotectiveness and social isolation. The family was Sikh and was isolated in a community that had only a small Sikh population. The mother's overprotectiveness was fueled by a driven husband whose work meant frequent absences. She appeared to keep her daughter close as an attempt to ward off her own depression.

This family's religious identity was a major factor in their social isolation; however, its members might have had similar difficulties were they not religious.

Seeing religious and spiritual factors as only social phenomena may seriously underestimate their influence. The worldview of many individuals is often the most important factor in their lives, with a key role in directing behavior, shaping relationships, and influencing attitudes toward their vocation.

Further, there is growing reason to see the spiritual as a dimension of experience—measurable in its own right and appropriate for interventions that are harmonized with those of clinical psychiatry and psychology. A "spiritual psychiatry" does not yet have markers analogous to the derangements of sleep, appetite, and sexual function that are assessed in biological psychiatry. Even so, Bergin suggested that "a spiritual conception of human nature which reorients personality theory" provides "a moral frame of reference for guiding and evaluating treatment procedures and outcomes and a developing body of spiritually derived interventions" (Bergin 1998, p. 6). This approach is in its infancy but is rapidly developing (Richards and Bergin 1997). Existential themes addressed by spiritual approaches include hope, identity, morality, meaning, and autonomy (see Chapter 4, "Therapeutic Implications of Worldview").

Finally, it may be important to distinguish spiritual phenomena from psychopathology. The self-absorption of clinical narcissism may be different but difficult to distinguish from the sin of pride. The scrupulosity and attention to detail of a devout religious believer may appear similar to the behavior of an obsessional patient. The guilt associated with depression may be distorted or may be related to actual misconduct about which the individual has strong feelings. Hopelessness may be a realistic response to real-life events or the fatalistic expression of an atheistic worldview. Both knowledge and clinical judgment are necessary to differentiate these perspectives, as is the humility to recognize that some phenomena may be better understood from a spiritual perspective.

Developing the Biopsychosociospiritual Formulation

The clinician who is interested in the interaction among risk and protective factors will want to explore if or how the patient's worldview has clinical relevance. The patient's worldview may not be particularly important, it may be one of several contributing variables to the onset of disorder, or it may be the most crucial variable. Determining the relative importance of each variable is the cornerstone of a useful formulation.

Much of medicine assumes the importance of interacting variables. For example, not all individuals with genetic vulnerability to schizophrenia develop the disorder. What protects those who are genetically vulnerable? Further, not all individuals who come from enmeshed, overprotective families develop anorexia nervosa. What protects some individuals from such a toxic family process?

Developmentalist Jerome Kagan (1988) summarized the interactive approach to formulations when he stated that "the stressfulness of an event depends on the psychobiologic surface upon which it strikes." Using this model, one would regard the patient's worldview as an element of his or her "psychobiologic" makeup. This interactionist view has been expressed differently by other developmentalists. Thomas and Chess (1980) described a "goodness of fit" occurring when the demands of the environment are balanced with the individual's abilities, style, and motivation. Within their framework, worldview could be seen as part of the motivational system of the individual.

A biopsychosociospiritual formulation can be seen as a type of mosaic, in which various risk and protective factors interact to form a clinical picture. For example, a dependent woman, genetically vulnerable to depression, is at increased risk for depressive affect if her emancipated children leave the home and her marriage is unsupportive. A child with a learning disorder is at increased risk if he or she is being raised by an economically challenged single parent in community with a resource-poor school system. Religious and spiritual factors fit similarly into the mosaic. A wife's terminal medical illness is even more distressing to a husband who views God as loving and supportive. A fundamentalist family may look to scriptures that address aspects of discipline to justify their controlling, even abusive, parenting practices.

By including worldview in this model of interacting risk and protective factors, the clinician comes to understand what behaviors and life events mean to the patient beyond their particular meaning based on the patient's internalized world of object relations. Knowledge of three areas is helpful in deciding how these meanings function in the patient's life: 1) ways that religion can function to promote or undermine health, 2) characteristics of the patient's particular tradition, and 3) psychiatric epidemiologic literature correlating measures of religion and spirituality with health.

Functions of Spirituality and Belief in Mental Health

There have been a number of attempts to distinguish levels of religious or spiritual maturity, health, and devotion. Perhaps the most widely known and utilized in research is the concept of intrinsic and extrinsic religiosity delineated by Allport and Ross (1967). Extrinsically religious individuals are those who use religion for social reasons, such as status and self-aggrandizement; intrinsically religious individuals internalize their beliefs and live them out regardless of the personal or external consequences. These individuals emphasize ends rather than means, and show unselfish, committed behavior rather than self-promoting behavior. Their expressed religious beliefs and spiritual values match their lifestyle and behavior. Research on religiosity can yield ambiguous results and obscure meaningful findings when it merges data from individuals with intrinsic religiosity with data from individuals with extrinsic religiosity.

However, even intrinsically held spiritual and other beliefs may be risk factors for the development or maintenance of psychopathology.

> A loving, supportive, religious family saw their child as special because he was a "gift from God." This theological view was recruited to support an indulging parenting pattern whereby their son was not held accountable for misconduct and did not develop mature coping capacities. His early adult life was plagued by termination of employment, failed interpersonal relationships, and substance abuse.

Most clinicians would agree that spirituality and religion can also function in healthy ways (Clinebell 1965; Malony 1985; Pargament 1997; Richards and Bergin 1997). Table 3–1 lists some healthy functions of spirituality and religion.

Evaluating a Particular Tradition or Belief System

To understand fully the role that worldview plays in a patient's life, one needs to understand something about the tradition associated with that worldview. For example, does the tradition in fact teach that any sexual pleasure outside of marriage is wrong? What does the patient's tradition or belief system say about how to deal with moral failure? Is there a range of interpretations of scripture within the patient's religious tradition (and, if so, has the patient selected among these interpretations)? Is unquestioning obedience to a leader required, suggesting that the patient may be part of a cult? Are there resources for emotional healing available in the congregation, such as pastoral counseling or small groups that meet for prayer? Consultation with an individual who is knowledgeable about the tradition may be necessary to learn the answers to these questions.

Spiritual and Religious Factors in Specific Disorders

For many years, scientific studies that explored etiologic factors in mental disorders neglected religious factors. Major psychiatric journals reported

TABLE 3–1.   Healthy functions of religion and spirituality

- Affirm relationships
- Strengthen basic trust in others specifically and in humankind generally
- Foster personal responsibility, including development of personal ethical guidelines
- Emphasize concern for others at a deeper level beyond surface behavior
- Enhance enjoyment of life through the appreciation of beauty, the encouragement of creativity, and other means
- Provide a flexible structure (i.e., rules) for life that encourages self-control and discipline and specifically facilitates the safe expression of sexuality and aggression
- Facilitate cognitive, emotional, and behavioral integration
- Provide an intellectual basis to manage doubt and difficult questions and thereby to manage existential anxiety
- Foster self-esteem and provide a sense of identity and ultimate worth
- Provide a sense of purpose and meaning that allows for rational interpretation of life's problems
- Demonstrate that love—and the positive emotions of hope, optimism, and peace—emerge from beliefs, rituals, and practices
- Offer a process of forgiveness and reconciliation that allows for the restoration and renewal of relationships
- Encourage the existence and maintenance of supportive community networks

Note: Each of these factors may *protect* individuals from the development of clinical problems. The converse of these characteristics or their absence may place individuals at *risk* for problems.

psychometric assessment of religion only rarely, and most studies that did assess religion examined only the variable of religious affiliation (Larson et al. 1986). Such single measures do not capture the multidimensional breadth of religion and spirituality, including aspects such as devotion and type of cognitive belief.

Several significant reviews of the relationship of religion and spirituality to health and mental health have emerged in the past decade (Koenig 1998; Koenig et al. 2001). Space limitations do not permit full discussion of these findings, but several are worth noting since they provide some data on which to base the development of individual formulations.

Depression

Kendler et al. (1997), in a large twin study based on data from the Virginia Twin Registry, noted that personal devotion buffered the effects of stressful life events on individuals prone to depression. A strong relationship between low levels of depression and high levels of personal religious devotion was found. Koenig et al. (1998a) described the effects of religious belief and activity on remission of depression in a group of medically ill hospitalized patients. They found that greater intrinsic religiosity independently predicted a shorter time to remission from depression. On the other hand, Koenig et al. (1998b) found that some types of religious coping were possibly associated with depression. The type of religious belief and coping that seemed to increase as depression symptoms increased included an image of God as punitive, the passive practicing of a religion, and being dissatisfied with one's own congregation.

Substance Abuse

Kendler et al. (1997) also reported on the relationship of religious devotion to substance abuse. They found that religious devotion was inversely correlated with current levels of alcohol use and lifetime risk for alcohol use. Studies of adolescents and young adults and studies of middle-aged and older populations consistently demonstrate an inverse relationship between substance abuse and religious involvement (Koenig et al. 2001). Potential mechanisms of this accepted relationship include the possibilities that religion and spirituality directly inculcate moral values that are protective, that the social support seen in religious and spiritual communities helps prevent social alienation, and that some increased psychological well-being in those who have a religious faith is protective against substance abuse. For some time, 12-step organizations have facilitated both spirituality and the maintenance of sobriety (Carroll 1993; Peteet 1993).

Anxiety Disorders

Freud viewed religion as an unrealistic attempt to escape anxiety, but more contemporary research suggests that religion can serve as a buffer against anxiety (Bergin 1983). Perhaps one of the more intriguing findings is that there appears to be a negative correlation between intrinsic religiousness and anxiety and a positive correlation between extrinsic religiousness and anxiety. Cross-cultural research on Christians and Buddhists supports this observation (Tapanya et al. 1997).

Child and Adolescent Disorders

Religious involvement of the family, as well as a teenager's religious commitment, plays an important role in delaying the onset of sexual intercourse with positive health consequences (Weaver et al. 2000). On the other hand, one study found that sexually active church-going teenage girls were less likely to use contraceptives than girls who were not church attendees, with the result that the church-going girls were at greater risk for unsafe sexual behavior and pregnancy (Studer and Thornton 1987). For some time, studies have consistently supported the position that religious beliefs and spiritual practices in the family and community are inversely related to antisocial behavior among youths. In one representative national study, Donahue and Benson (1995) reported that religious involvement among youths was associated with less likelihood of trouble with police, fighting, vandalism, and physical assault. Finally, family stressors such as marital conflict and divorce have consistently been linked with adverse mental health outcomes in children. Several studies have shown an association between spiritual or religious involvement and a supportive, cohesive family environment (Mahoney et al. 2001). On the other hand, while a preponderance of research evidence has emphasized the benefits of spirituality in children's mental health, some studies show negative effects of religion and spirituality, in particular through the condoning of harshness and rigidity, the converse of structure and support (Sorenson et al. 1995).

Relationships Between Religious and Spiritual Problems and Mental Disorders

How does the process of formulation relate to current diagnostic practice? Religious and spiritual factors can be coded in two ways in the DSM nomenclature; these categorizations reflect several types of directional effects.

Religious and spiritual problems may be a focus of clinical attention in individuals who do or do not have mental disorders, and the DSM-IV-TR contains a V code for treating distress associated with a spiritual or religious problem (V62.89) (American Psychiatric Association 2000, p. 741). The V code can be used concomitantly with other diagnoses when they coexist.

Axis IV in DSM-IV-TR, which describes psychosocial and environmental problems, provides a second place to classify religious and spiritual problems that do not meet the threshold for a V code. According to DSM-IV-TR, a psychosocial or environmental problem can play a role "in the initiation or exacerbation of a mental disorder" (be a cause) and may also "develop as a consequence of a person's psychopathology" (be an effect) (American Psychiatric Association 2000; p. 31). Similarly, a patient's spiritual or religious problems or worldview may predispose the patient to psychopathology or may be a consequence of psychopathology.

Turner and colleagues (1995) identified several types of spiritual and religious problems. Religious problems could include conversion to a new religion (including cults), a rejection of a prior religion or loss of faith, the intensification of beliefs and practices, and experiences of guilt. Spiritual problems may include mystical experiences, near-death experiences, and re-actions to terminal illness. Two core areas of human concern—moral and ex-istential—must always be considered as potential sources of problems. Clinicians have traditionally dealt with neurotic guilt but have had less clear ways of dealing with guilt that results from actual offenses that a patient committed. Further, changes in one's family relationships, vocational rela-tionships, and health status often lead patients to ask ultimate questions. Questioning can engender dysphoria and hopelessness as components of existential despair. The following case vignettes illustrate various ways that problems related to spirituality, religion, and worldview can present clinically.

Moral concerns, including moral failure or a moral dilemma, can be as-sociated with significant distress:

A 52-year-old woman was finally apprehended for her role as an accomplice in a murder many years earlier. She described relief at shedding her assumed identity, and she related that guilt, anxiety, and depression had plagued her for years as she harbored the knowledge of her wrongdoing. She described several trials of antidepressant therapy as well as psychotherapy that had been unsuccessful. Her arrest and legal accountability resulted in relief of her symptoms.

A 36-year-old married mother of two presented with a 3-month history of sleeplessness, decreased appetite, and tearfulness. In describing the vegeta-tive signs of depression, she noted that her husband of 11 years had recently left her and their two children for another woman. The patient described sadness and anger at her situation and was particularly full of rage when she stated that "my kids are being hurt."

In each of these cases, behavior that would be considered a moral transgres-sion in most religious traditions caused enough distress to bring patients to psychiatric attention. What they believed about guilt and forgiveness was important in formulating an understanding of their distress. Sheehan and Kroll (1990) reported that numerous patients seen in a mental health con-text believed they had done something wrong that had led to their condition, a finding that was not explained by psychosis or depression.

An unhealthy religious environment and the distorted use of theology or an agnostic worldview can contribute to mental disorder, as shown in the following examples:

A 15-year-old girl was admitted to a psychiatric ward after a suicide attempt. Family evaluation revealed a tense relationship between the girl and her fa-ther, an elder in a conservative Protestant denomination. The emotional re-strictiveness of the family, particularly in rejecting her interest in a male who did not attend their church, led to significant anger. The teenager com-

plained of her parents' hypocrisy: "They preach love but are very unaccept-
ing people." The teenager attempted suicide after her mother tried to read
her diary.

This adolescent's religious family was well meaning but believed that structure for their daughter meant excessive control of her activities. Their use of
conservative theology alienated her further.

> A 45-year-old Christian hospital social worker presented for evaluation and
> treatment of depressive symptoms. Before the evaluation, he had become in-
> creasingly burdened with his responsibilities and the fact that there were so
> many needy people that "I can't help." His developmental history revealed
> that he was a peacemaker in his home, where there had been considerable
> parental conflict. He described having been controlling in personal relation-
> ships and always trying to "make things right." When situations were out of
> his control, he tried even harder to make his immediate relationships peace-
> ful. He often felt anxious and guilty that he couldn't do more for others. He
> stated that "I would give up my satisfaction for the peace of others," yet he
> acknowledged that such subservience made him full of rage. As therapy pro-
> ceeded, he began to accept that he could not "solve all the world's problems"
> and that the excessive expectations he placed on himself frequently triggered
> his dysphoria. He attributed his giving tendencies to his beliefs about what
> it meant to be a Christian, which, through therapy and consultation with
> clergy, he came to realize were distorted. With time he came to see that he
> could still be the giving, loving person he believed he should be—crucial
> aspects of his professional and religious identity—yet also "take care of
> myself."

This self-effacing and introspective social worker was subservient to others
yet was angry when he behaved in this manner. This anger was not consistent with his view of Christian servanthood. His therapist needed to discuss
with him whether this view was an accurate interpretation of his faith's
teachings, and he referred the patient to his pastor for further clarification of
this issue.

> A 62-year-old successful businessman first came to the psychiatry clinic be-
> cause of problems with his stepson from his third marriage. He was estranged
> from his older two children. He had had no prior psychiatric treatment but
> described a lack of energy and general hopelessness for the future, although
> he was not suicidal. In a marital session in which his stepson was discussed,
> he volunteered the following material.
>
> Therapist: "The last time we met, you mentioned something that inter-
> ested me. You stated that you weren't optimistic about people. Could you tell
> me more?"
>
> Patient: "Yeah, I'll tell you how I see it. Over 2,500 years ago, a group of
> people got together in the desert and said, 'We can't take each other's goats
> any more and keep raping each other's wives. We've got to stop this and have

some rules.' So Yahweh from Mt. Sinai came up with some rules, and these people began to use them. It kind of kept things under control for them. But, you know what, whenever you prick the bubble, lots of darkness and evil spill out. When the lights are out and it's dark, what happens? I'll tell you what happens. Nothing good happens. People do things that they don't want seen, and the overwhelming majority of people are like this.... I talked with a very powerful political leader lately, one who is a leader in our community. I asked him, 'Would you give up all your power if all the children could be cured of cancer—children in the world?' He kind of smiled at me, and I'll tell you what the smile meant—'No, I would never give up that power for anything'—and all people are like that. I've been done in by business many times. You can't be naive to survive out there."

In this example, as the treating clinician asked a question meant to probe for depressive symptoms and possible failed relationships, the patient's cynicism and hopelessness emerged. These characteristics seemed to be both fueled by and a consequence of his agnosticism and his conflicted attitude toward religion and spirituality.

When religious and spiritual problems both result from and complicate psychiatric disorders, they may require vigorous intervention:

> A 37-year-old single woman presented with symptoms of anxiety, depression, excessive anger, and poor impulse control. One of eight children born to a conservative Catholic family, she had difficulty becoming emancipated from the family. Her anxiety, depression, and "inner emptiness" had been associated with intermittent excessive alcohol use and numerous sexual relationships, and she had required psychiatric admission 13 times over the course of 4 years.
>
> She related to her therapist that earlier in her life, in the context of promiscuity and alcohol use, she had become pregnant and had an abortion. This experience was associated with severe guilt and rumination that she had committed an unpardonable sin. At the time of reconsultation, her guilt and sense of alienation from a church that would no longer accept her appeared to be more clinically prominent than her pervasive low self-esteem. Unable to rejoin her spiritual community as a result of her sexual behavior, she felt increasingly isolated.

This woman's developmental and personality difficulties contributed to behavior that caused her considerable secondary religious and spiritual distress.

Sometimes a religious and spiritual problem has an even more complex relationship to an individual's psychiatric disorder:

> A successful lawyer in the middle stage of his career received a significant employment opportunity with a prestigious law firm, a change that required his family to move. His 16-year-old daughter, who had a diagnosis of anorexia nervosa, had recently recovered from a protracted episode of weight loss

and did not want to move. She also had "become more spiritual" and begun daily meditation. In consultation with his daughter's psychiatrist, who suggested that a move might not be in his daughter's best interest, her father stated, "Sometimes you just have to climb the mountain." A review of his religious history suggested a background of nominal Catholicism. His career was one in which advancement, secular success, and financial achievement were prominent. His wife was somewhat depressed about his decision and asked him, "What's really important in life, anyway?"

This patient's narcissistic behavior coexisted with a type of functional agnosticism, both of which were important in understanding his case.

The following two case vignettes also demonstrate how religious and spiritual issues are intertwined with the individual's problem and his or her family:

A 16-year-old boy was seen for conduct problems. In the process of psychotherapy and behavioral management training, his parents requested a marital session with the psychiatrist. They described difficulties in their relationship and substance abuse on the husband's part. The husband was the son of a minister who had extremely high expectations and as a perfectionist offered very little praise to his children. When the couple had an unplanned pregnancy before being married, the husband had experienced harsh rejection from his family of origin, and his father had demanded that they abort the child. The couple described their longstanding anger toward the husband's father and, at the same time, described being in a new parish where their spiritual needs were being met. In this instance, the family history suggested that the influence of distorted and harsh religious ideas were a risk factor in the husband's development, but the current religious community was an asset to marital and family stability.

A 22-year-old premedical student revealed to his educational counselor that his interest in philosophical themes and his belief that religion is "not scientific" had resulted in an estrangement between him and his religious family. He expressed a longing for a closer relationship with his family, but he had no specific psychiatric symptoms. In this situation, the patient's spiritual problem and distress were not associated with a clinical condition and occurred in the absence of a mental disorder.

In constructing a biopsychosociospiritual formulation, a clinician will be using information from the religious and spiritual assessment to decide whether the patient's beliefs and practices have a healthy (integrating and positive) versus a pathological (fragmenting and distressing) role in the patient's life and presenting problems (Gabbard et al. 1982). At times a patient's beliefs and practices may seem unusual. For example, glossolalia, which is a state of excited utterance of religious significance to certain groups that emphasize emotional types of spiritual experience, may appear to be a type of manic excitement. At times religious ideation can be part of psychotic behavior, as in the case of the murder defendant who stated that God told him to cut the throat of a young boy. In similar instances, the clinician can usually recognize that pathology fits common patterns of mental illness, that the pathological behavior is not shared by others of the same faith, and that most religious perspectives would not support behavior of extreme destructiveness. In challenging cases, a clinician may need to consult with clergy or a proponent of the patient's worldview.

Chapter 1, "Introduction: Definition and Significance of a Worldview," and Chapters 5–10, on separate faith traditions, illustrate that a clinician's own worldview has a significant effect on clinical practice. Even a clinician who is technically neutral in conducting assessments and treatments has a worldview. Clinicians can either overidentify with a religious position or reject it as a problem, for example, as a type of wish fulfillment. Unless these tendencies are carefully monitored, the clinician's worldview can complicate the difficult tasks of distinguishing realistic guilt for a moral transgression from pathological guilt and distinguishing healthy, religiously inspired altruism from unhealthy, self-defeating masochism (Gartner et al. 1990).

A clinician's worldview has its own unique developmental dynamics. Just as a religiously conservative clinician may have "blind spots," an atheistic clinician needs to be aware of tendencies that are influenced by his or her worldview. Research indicates that both belief and disbelief, manifested by one's internal object representations of God, are influenced by relationships with parental figures (Rizzuto 1979). This internal "psychospiritual" cognitive set will strongly influence clinical work and needs to be handled in the same manner as any countertransference phenomenon (Abernethy and Lancia 1998).

Summary

Spiritual factors and philosophical beliefs may contribute to psychopathology and may also promote health. The challenge of formulating a given case is to clarify the interaction of these factors with biological, psychological, and social factors. Doing so may require the clinician to examine the influence of his or her own worldview and to research the beliefs and resources of unfamiliar traditions. A solid biopsychosociospiritual formulation is the basis of effective treatment.

References

Abernethy AD, Lancia JJ: Religion and the psychotherapeutic relationship: transferential and countertransferential dimensions. J Psychother Pract Res 7:281–289, 1998

Allport GW, Ross JM: Personal religious orientation and prejudice. J Pers Soc Psychol 5:432–443, 1967

American Psychiatric Association: Diagnostic and Statistical Manual of Mental Disorders , 4th Edition, Text Revision. Washington, DC, American Psychiatric Association, 2000

Bergin AE: Religiosity and mental health: a critical reevaluation and meta-analysis. Prof Psychol Res Pract 14:170–184, 1983

Bergin AE: Religion and mental health: spiritual and religious issues in psychopathology and psychotherapy (Oskar Pfister Award Lecture). Paper presented at the annual meeting of the American Psychiatric Association, Toronto, ON, Canada, May 30–June 4, 1998

Carroll S: Spirituality and purpose in life in alcoholism recovery. J Stud Alcohol 54:297–301, 1993

Clinebell HJ Jr: Mental Health Through Christian Community. Nashville, TN, Abingdon Press, 1965

Donahue MJ, Benson PL: Religion and the well-being of adolescents. J Soc Issues 51:145–160, 1995

Engel GL: The need for a new medical model: a challenge for biomedicine. Science 196:129–136, 1977

Engel GL: The clinical application of the biopsychosocial model. Am J Psychiatry 137:535–544, 1980

Gabbard GO, Twemlow SW, Jones FC: Differential diagnosis of altered mind/body perception. Psychiatry 45:361–369, 1982

Gartner J, Harmatz M, Hohmann A, et al: The effects of patient and clinician ideology on clinical judgment: a study of ideological countertransference. Psychotherapy 27:98–104, 1990

Kagan J: Stress and coping in early development, in Stress, Coping, and Development in Children. Edited by Garmezy N, Rutter M. Baltimore, MD, Johns Hopkins University Press, 1988, pp 191–216

Kendler KS, Gardner CO, Prescott CA: Religion, psychopathology, and substance abuse: a multimeasure, genetic-epidemiologic study. Am J Psychiatry 154:322–329, 1997

Koenig HG (ed): Handbook of Religion and Mental Health. San Diego, CA, Academic Press, 1998

Koenig HG, George LK, Peterson BL: Religiosity and remission of depression in medically ill older patients. Am J Psychiatry 155:536–542, 1998a

Koenig, HG, Pargament KI, Nielsen J: Religious coping and health status in medically ill hospitalized older adults. J Nerv Ment Dis 186:513–521, 1998b

Koenig HG, McCullough ME, Larson DB: Handbook of Religion and Health. New York, Oxford University Press, 2001

Larson DB, Pattison EM, Blazer DG, et al: Systematic analysis of research on religious variables in four major psychiatric journals, 1978–1982. Am J Psychiatry 143:329–334, 1986

Mahoney A, Pargament KI, Tarakeshwar N, et al: Religion in the home in the 1980s and 1990s: a meta-analytic review and conceptual analysis of links between religion, marriage, and parenting. J Family Psychol 15:559–596, 2001

Malony HN: Assessing religious maturity, in Psychotherapy and the Religiously Committed Patient. Edited by Stern EM. New York, Haworth Press, 1985, pp 25–33

Pargament KI: The Psychology of Religion and Coping: Theory, Research, Practice. New York, Guilford, 1997

Peteet JR: A closer look at the role of a spiritual approach in addictions treatment. J Subst Abuse Treat 10:263–267, 1993

Richards PS, Bergin A: Spiritual Strategy for Counseling and Psychotherapy. Washington, DC, American Psychological Association, 1997

Rizzuto AM: The Birth of the Living God: A Psychoanalytic Inquiry. Chicago, IL, University of Chicago Press, 1979

Sheehan W, Kroll J: Psychiatric patients' belief in general health factors and sin as causes of illness. Am J Psychiatry 147:112–113, 1990

Sorenson AM, Grindstaff CF, Turner RJ: Religious involvement among unmarried adolescent mothers: a source of emotional support? Sociol Relig 56:71–81, 1995

Studer M, Thornton A: Adolescent religiosity and contraceptive usage. J Marriage Fam 49:117–128, 1987

Tapanya S, Nicki R, Jarusawad O: Worry and intrinsic/extrinsic religious orientation among Buddhist (Thai) and Christian (Canadian) elderly persons. Int J Aging Hum Dev 44:73–83, 1997

Thomas A, Chess S: The Dynamics of Psychological Development. New York, Brunner/Mazel, 1980

Turner RP, Lukoff D, Barnhouse RT, et al: Religious or spiritual problem: a culturally sensitive diagnostic category in the DSM-IV. J Nerv Ment Dis 183:435–444, 1995

Weaver AJ, Samford JA, Morgan V, et al: Research on religious variables in five major adolescent research journals: 1992 to 1996. J Nerv Ment Dis 188:36–44, 2000

CHAPTER 4

Therapeutic Implications of Worldview

John R. Peteet, M.D.

Clinicians increasingly agree that they should appreciate the diversity of their patients' cultural and religious beliefs (Koenig 1998; Richards and Bergin 2000). But what importance should these beliefs have in treatment? When and how does a therapist's own worldview matter? This chapter briefly explores the relevance of worldview in the treatment of patients with existential concerns—specifically concerns about identity, hope, meaning and purpose, morality, and relationship to authority. It then distinguishes four general approaches to such problems and reviews the ethical challenges of dealing explicitly with worldviews in the role of a therapist.

Beliefs have emerged as an important focus of clinical attention. Patients' expectations and assumptions powerfully enhance trust and influence treatment outcome (Benson 1996; Frank 1991). Addressing faulty beliefs that underlie the maladaptive patterns may be central in both cognitive-behavioral and dynamically oriented psychotherapy (Wright et al. 2003; Horowitz 1991). Furthermore, therapists bring their own values and beliefs to the treatment situation (Kluft 1992; Schafer 1970). Beliefs about the nature of reality are particularly germane when working within the domain where clinical and existential concerns overlap (Figure 4–1).

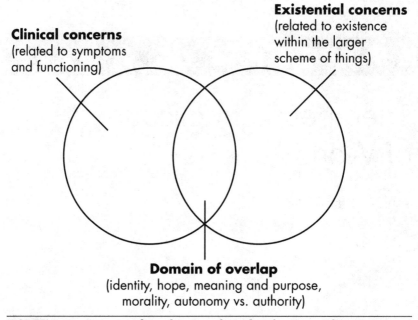

Clinical concerns
(related to symptoms
and functioning)

Existential concerns
(related to existence
within the larger
scheme of things)

Domain of overlap
(identity, hope, meaning and purpose,
morality, autonomy vs. authority)

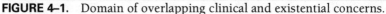

FIGURE 4–1.   Domain of overlapping clinical and existential concerns.

Working with Existential Concerns in the Clinical Setting

Identity

Identity is especially important at points of change, such as the transition of an immigrant to a new culture. Similarly, the transition to adulthood may cause an adolescent to struggle with who she wants to be. A businessman recovering from a heart attack may wonder if he is the same person. And a recovering cocaine addict who realizes how she has neglected her children's needs may question what kind of person she has become. For answers to such questions people often turn to their core beliefs: "I may not be what I thought I was (or should be), but I know I am loved, or worthwhile because …(e.g., I believe in being a devoted parent, or because God loves me)." These beliefs may have childhood roots in the patient's worldview or cultural identity or may reflect a new identity. The lives of Malcolm X and Charles Colson are recent examples of how dramatic changes in worldviews can follow major life changes.

Patients sometimes want therapists to help them understand whether their core beliefs (e.g., that they deserve punishment) are distorted by emotional factors such as depression. They may also struggle with the implications of a religious identity ("Does being a faithful Catholic mean that I need to accept how my husband treats me?"). They may also be actively comparing their own worldview with alternatives that promise a different identity.

To help patients with such concerns, therapists first need to convey that the patient's worldview is respected, if not shared.

> A 45-year-old separated architect and father of three came for treatment because he felt torn about coming out as a gay man. In addition to feeling responsible for his family, he had religious reservations about practicing homosexuality that he felt were being dismissed as homophobic prejudices by his therapist at a gay and lesbian treatment center. As a Christian who had never regularly attended church, he did not have a pastor. Instead, he sought out a therapist who shared his religious worldview in the hope that the therapist could help him integrate his religious and gender identities. After meeting with the therapist for several months, he became more comfortable about moving in with a male partner. He consulted the therapist again at times when he felt undecided about his obligations toward his children or about how well his behavior was matching his ideals.

The therapist in this case acknowledged but never explicitly discussed his own worldview, and the therapist never suggested that the patient change his own worldview. Their shared religious identification functioned primarily to reassure the patient that his moral and religious commitments were being taken seriously. In other cases, a therapist might approach a patient in ways that reflect more clearly the influence of the therapist's own worldview. For example, an atheist who values autonomy highly might ask a patient in search of direction, "Who or what do you want to be?" A Jewish therapist who sees identity as rooted in a larger context may ask, "Who are you in relation to your community and commitments?" And a Christian therapist who sees identity as formed in response to moral and spiritual challenges (recalling that Jesus said, "The person who saves his life will lose it") may ask, "Who do you feel called to be?"

Patients also identify with qualities in the therapist that are informed by the therapist's worldview—for example, a Buddhist's compassion or an atheist's skeptical honesty.

Hope

Cognitive approaches are useful in treating anxiety and depressive disorders because hope is so often tied to beliefs. When loss or serious illness shakes a religious person's belief in God, he or she can become cynical or may experience despair.

> A 26-year-old graduate student presented with depression and suicidal thoughts after breaking off his engagement. He had met his fiancée through

an evangelical student organization, and her enthusiastic faith assuaged his concerns about her past relationships with a number of men. However, when he discovered that she had lied to him repeatedly about previous relationships, he felt not only disillusioned with her but betrayed by God. Treatment involved helping him to reexamine his faith and what it taught him about the nature of the divine.

People who instead ground their ultimate hopes in transcendent ideals such as compassion, truth, or justice may also be vulnerable to despair if they are disillusioned by important figures in their lives.

A 30-year-old physicist became seriously depressed after his father, who was a successful academic, died of alcoholism. The patient had rejected his family's Catholicism as rigid and naive and instead committed himself to truth and the scientific method. Later, when he saw his laboratory chief and mentor behave in self-serving ways, he began to doubt whether honesty and integrity existed and whether science could lead to a significantly better world. He spent considerable time in treatment expressing these doubts and thinking through why he should go on living.

Disillusionment with his father and later with his boss darkened this patient's view of the world, and the loss of his ideals further diminished his hope. Overcoming his cynicism required him to both grieve these losses and to reformulate his view of the world.

Patients who are confronting death often draw hope from their worldview. For example, Christians believe in the "sure and certain hope of resurrection," and Hindus in reincarnation. Some suicidal patients entertain fantasies of reunion with loved ones after death; many report being deterred from certain actions by fear of punishment in the next life.

A therapist can influence his or her patient's search for ultimate hope in several ways. He or she can empathize with the patient's questions, point out the distorting effects of despair on the clarity of the patient's perspective, and help the patient consider whether to consult other possible sources of answers, such as a pastor. A therapist of the same faith can sometimes go further in "lending" a patient hope by affirming the hope that their shared worldview offers (the clinical, transference, countertransference, and boundary aspects of taking on this role are discussed later in this chapter).

Meaning and Purpose

Many individuals bring into treatment their search for purpose and the larger meaning of their suffering (Herman 1992; Yalom 1980). An atheist who loses a child to cancer may question whether his life has any purpose. A trauma survivor who is religious may question whether he can continue to believe that God is fair or loving (Peteet 2001). A depressed patient who loses his job may fear that he is being punished for an unpardonable sin.

The therapist can sometimes help a patient bring to bear the perspective offered by the patient's worldview—for example, a Buddhist's emphasis on compassion and detachment, a Muslim's on reverence, a Christian's on grace, an atheist's on realism or autonomy, and a secular humanist's on service.

> A hospital psychiatrist saw in consultation a 60-year-old retired Unitarian minister with colon cancer who had depression and suicidal ideation. The patient explained, "If I believed there were an authority out there taking care of things to whom I was responsible, I would feel differently, but I don't. I simply believe in service. When I can't continue to improve things, what's the point of going on?"
>
> The psychiatrist explored why the patient's recent incapacitation seemed to have invalidated a life of service and his worth to family and friends. Did his liberal, humanistic worldview require this conclusion, or was his counterdependent personality the more important factor? Rather than focusing on the relationship between his counterdependence and his vulnerability to depression if he did not consider himself "productive," the psychiatrist drew his attention to ways in which the patient's giving others the opportunity to serve him had given his life meaning and could continue to do so.

Although Propst et al. (1992) have shown that religiously based cognitive therapy can be effective in treating depression even when conducted by nonreligious therapists, therapists who share their patients' spiritual commitment are often better able to help them find the meaning offered by belief in a transcendent reality (Richards and Bergin 1997). However, the therapist's worldview may be brought into therapy in inappropriate or coercive ways—as, for example, when a conservative Christian therapist suggests praying with a patient or an atheistic therapist tells a recently born-again Christian patient that he or she is "too religious."

Morality

A patient's religious and philosophical beliefs influence how he or she functions morally in several ways. Beliefs about the nature of God and of the moral universe shape a person's commitments to justice, caring, honesty, and other values. Philosophical or religious ways of thinking (e.g., reliance on authority or reliance on free thought) guide the way people make moral decisions. For example, in choosing a career or a partner, some individuals seek God's will, while others seek the integrity that comes from living consistently with their own highest values and beliefs. Religious traditions both articulate standards of right and wrong and offer options for dealing with moral failure (e.g., confession, forgiveness, making amends). Twelve-step traditions and several religious traditions encourage confession and surrender to a higher power, and approaches such as Albert Ellis's rational emotive therapy (and that of Smart Recovery, the program for substance abusers to which it gave rise) emphasize rational self-reliance (Rational-Emotive Behavior Therapy 2004; Smart Recovery 2004). Faith-based communities and service organizations help support virtues that are central to clinical work, including integrity, equanimity, humility, honesty, and caring.

Patients who are trying to make an accurate assessment of their guilt may need help distinguishing their tradition's teaching about a particular behavior from their own emotion-laden interpretation of those teachings. Does the church or the tradition's scriptures teach that experiencing any sexual pleasure outside of marriage is wrong, or is this interpretation a manifestation of the patient's depression? A therapist engaged in helping a patient who is struggling with controversial issues, including the morality of homosexuality or abortion, may need to assist the patient in appreciating the range of beliefs about these issues held by others who hold the patient's worldview (Haldeman 1996).

A clinician's values inevitably influence those of his or her patients (Kelly and Strupp 1992) and the approach the clinician takes to moral dilemmas in treatment. A religious therapist who is committed to marital fidelity may work harder to prevent a divorce and to find avenues to reconciliation in its aftermath than one whose worldview places a higher value on freedom of choice.

Autonomy and Authority

The worldviews of religious and nonreligious individuals differ most sharply on the question of ultimate authority. Secularists will often grant the usefulness of religious belief, if only as a crutch, for a patient who seeks meaning or hope, but they more often see problems with many religions' insistence on obedience to authority. Atheists value freedom from obedience to an authority outside of the natural universe. For example, Freud, an atheist, saw psychoanalysis as a way to help individuals overcome their neurotic dependence on religion. By contrast, clinicians with a religious worldview value enhancement of freedom to help patients realize not only their own goals within a natural ecosystem but their place within a created order. A therapist's vision of what it means for human beings to flourish is inevitably (if only implicitly) informed by what his or her faith tradition teaches about human nature, relatedness, fallibility, and redemption. For example, a religious clinician will tend to respond to a request for assisted suicide by giving weight not only to autonomy but to other considerations such as respect for life, the meaning of relatedness, and the physician's role as healer (Meier et al. 1998; Portenoy et al. 1997). He or she will want to treat problems such as depression and anxiety not only because they cause suffering but also because they interfere with living fully within the context of who the patient was created to be.

> A married secretary in her late 30s came to a therapist requesting help in deciding what to do about an affair she had begun with her boss. She reported feeling guilty because "the nuns in my Catholic school always told me this was wrong." On the other hand, she found her marriage unsatisfying and her husband "boring."

Both an atheistic and a religious therapist might explore how this patient understands her tradition's precepts about marriage and what factors contribute to her ambivalence. However, while a therapist who views these precepts as arbitrary and rigid might try to help her become freer of their influence, a religiously committed therapist would be more apt to discuss how the patient understands and integrates these precepts with her obligations to her husband and to God. A religiously committed therapist might also think about referring the patient to a pastoral counselor who could help her consider how her tradition stands on these questions.

Similarly, religious and nonreligious therapists tend to have contrasting approaches to autonomy as expressed in the issues of assisted suicide, abortion, adolescent sex, and homosexuality.

> The Evangelical Protestant parents of a 12-year-old girl who was being treated for depression and poor school performance discovered that she had begun to experiment sexually with a 14-year-old classmate. Their daughter's therapist was a lapsed Catholic who saw her task as helping the patient to think for herself. Accordingly, she focused with the patient on the choice of what to do with her body, advised the parents to have her see a pediatrician to discuss birth control, and expressed concern about the dangers of making the patient feel overly ashamed of her behavior. Her parents took the contrasting position (consistent with their worldview) that they should exert their authority to prevent the patient from acting on her sexual impulses until she was considerably older and more mature.
>
> This therapist's emphasis on promoting autonomy and minimizing shame had developed in part in reaction to what she felt was an authoritarian Catholic upbringing. After it became clear how much her belief contrasted with the parents' commitment to having their daughter become more connected and responsible to a caring ultimate authority, they agreed that the patient should see a different therapist who could support their efforts to parent her in ways that were more consistent with their religious worldview.

Four Approaches to Concerns Involving Worldview

How should a therapist deal explicitly with a patient's spiritual or philosophical concerns—for example, a patient's crisis of faith or religious objections to taking medication? (See the DSM-IV-TR V code for religious or spiritual problem [American Psychiatric Association 2000, p. 741].) A number of factors are relevant, including the patient's primary need (e.g., growth vs. help with adjustment or problem solving) and the nature, specific aims, and timing of the work (e.g., psychological insight into a maladaptive pattern vs. resolution of a conflict). These factors in turn influence the degree of direct support needed and the amount of interpersonal closeness that is appropriate. Additional factors include the importance of spiritual factors in the patient's life, the patient's presenting problems and attitude toward treatment, the interest of the patient to integrate psychological perspectives with other perspectives, the availability of outside philosophical or spiritual resources, and the therapist's own knowledge and preferred style (Table 4–1).

TABLE 4–1.   Four approaches to concerns involving worldview in clinical practice

---

- Acknowledge the problem, but limit discussion to its psychological dimension.

- Clarify the aspects of the problem that involve worldview as well as the problem's psychological dimensions, offer the patient suggestions for dealing with the problematic aspects of his or her worldview, and consider working with an outside resource, such as a religious community or other authority.

- Address the problem indirectly by using the patient's own philosophy of life.

- Address the problem directly by using a shared perspective.

Depending on the nature of these factors, a therapist might choose one of four approaches (Peteet 1994). In the most familiar and straightforward of these approaches, the therapist **acknowledges the problem but limits discussion to its psychological dimension.** For example, the therapist might address a patient's anger at God by examining the patient's relationship with other authority figures in his life.

A second possible approach would be to **clarify the worldview as well as the psychological aspects of the problem, suggest resources to help the patient deal with the problematic aspects of his or her worldview, and consider working with an outside resource,** such as a religious community or other authority. This approach might include enlisting a hospital chaplain or clergyperson to offer spiritual help or referring the patient to a therapist who shares the patient's religious or spiritual tradition. It could also involve referral to organized programs that integrate beliefs and emotions, including religiously or spiritually based cognitive-behavioral therapy (Bilu et al 1993; Propst et al. 1992) or 12-step programs.

In a third approach, the therapist would have the aim of **addressing the** problem indirectly by using the patient's own philosophy of life. This approach might include exploring ways the patient can make better use of his or her resources and tradition (e.g., by examining a range of beliefs within the patient's own denomination or examining misconceptions about the spiritual nature of Alcoholics Anonymous).

A fourth approach would be to **address the problem directly together by using a shared perspective.** The basis for this approach could range from the therapist's agreement with the patient about the importance of hope, meaning, worldview, or a caring community to the prescriptive use of shared values, beliefs, or practices (e.g., meditation or scripture) in the treatment. The fourth approach requires particularly careful attention to transference and countertransference and to boundary and consent issues.

Ethical Challenges in Dealing Explicitly With Worldview Issues

Transference and Countertransference

Patients often develop transference responses to therapists based on their perception of the therapist's worldview. For example, patients who believe (or suspect, for example, on the basis of the therapist's last name) that the therapist shares their worldview may unconsciously respond to the therapist on the basis of their formative experiences with religious figures. They may be more likely to trust a therapist who understands and shares important values and beliefs, or they may be ashamed to share their moral failings with a therapist of the same faith. Attempts to discuss the implications of their worldview for their problems or concerns can lead to unproductive arguments if these discussions revive earlier struggles with religious authorities. In addition, a patient who knows or assumes that a therapist has a different worldview can either suspect the therapist of undermining cherished values or regard the therapist as a safer and more objective counselor than someone from the patient's own tradition.

Countertransference responses also differ depending on whether the patient and therapist share the same worldview. For example, a therapist who is treating a patient who shares the therapist's tradition may respond to the patient's conservatism by reacting as he did to his fundamentalist father's conservatism or may attempt to enlighten a younger patient with whom he identifies. A therapist of a patient from a different tradition may unconsciously recoil from religious beliefs the therapist finds personally repugnant.

Transference and countertransference interactions related to worldview may be complementary (e.g., parent and child or teacher and seeker), merging (e.g., as when a sense of religious intimacy leads to avoidance of needed confrontation), oppositional (e.g., with engagement of old conflicts with religious authority), or nuanced in even more complex ways (Abernethy and Lancia 1998).

Boundaries

More than clinicians in other medical specialties, psychotherapists need to think about the meaning of a patient's question. The clinical context sometimes dictates that a patient's question be explored and sometimes that it be answered directly. When does devoting clinical attention to questions of morality, meaning, or worldview violate acceptable boundaries of psychotherapy? Is it ever appropriate for a therapist to discuss his or her own worldview? Should one ever treat a member of one's own congregation or agree to pray or discuss scripture with a patient? Partly because of concerns about the abuse of such practices, the American Psychiatric Association (1990) approved a set of guidelines regarding possible conflict between religious commitments and psychiatric practice. The guidelines remind clinicians that they must maintain respect for their patients' beliefs and that they should neither impose their own religious, antireligious, or ideological beliefs on their patients nor substitute such beliefs for accepted diagnostic concepts or therapeutic practice.

Gutheil and Gabbard (1993, 1998) distinguished between "boundary crossing," a descriptive term, and "boundary violation," which represents a harmful crossing or transgression of a boundary. As they noted, the specific effect of a boundary crossing can be assessed only by careful attention to the clinical context. Suggesting prayer in therapy may be coercive and unethical, but, depending on the clinical context, it may be therapeutic to accept a patient's request to pray together if the therapist can do so sincerely and with a clear understanding of how it advances the goals of the psychotherapy.

Given the power differential between the therapist and the patient, attention to such boundaries will always be necessary. At the same time, clinicians should work to reduce this power differential by encouraging more mutual relationships in therapy (Blackshaw and Miller 1994). As the Massachusetts Board of Registration in Medicine's 1994 guidelines related to boundaries in psychotherapy point out, self-disclosure should generally be kept to a minimum in psychotherapy, but self-disclosure is appropriate on some occasions (e.g., discussion of the physician's training and qualifications), and on infrequent occasions self-disclosure can have a significant therapeutic impact (Commonwealth of Massachusetts 1994). The guidelines state, "These situations need to be well thought out, and it must be clear that these disclosures serve the patient, not the therapist" (Commonwealth of Massachusetts 1994, p. 4).

A therapist who is asked to see a fellow congregant as a patient should seriously consider the potential effect of their kinship in faith on the therapeutic relationship and should explore its meaning. Will the patient trust only a therapist who is a fellow congregant? Is the patient seeking to avoid an issue through establishing a special connection with the therapist? If the patient is being referred by a respected figure in the church hierarchy, will the therapist feel pressure to treat the patient differently? Anticipating and discussing these issues and maintaining confidentiality are particularly important in considering therapy for a fellow congregant.

Few data are available about how therapists influence patients on the basis of their own worldviews or how often therapists use religious interventions such as prayer or scripture reading in psychotherapy. In one of the few existing studies of such practices, Galanter et al. (1991) surveyed 193 psychiatrist members of the Christian Medical and Dental Society and found that about half of the respondents said they would discourage strongly religious patients from getting an abortion or engaging in homosexual acts or premarital sex, and about one-third said they would discourage other patients from these activities. Whether a patient was committed to Christian beliefs made a significant difference in whether the respondents would recommend prayer to the patient. These findings suggest that at least some religious therapists choose the fourth approach discussed earlier (dealing with spiritual problems by using a shared worldview). More research is needed on the boundary implications of this approach.

Consent

Finally, patient-therapist differences in worldview can make informed consent centrally important. Because the therapist him- or herself constitutes the therapeutic instrument, the therapist must make his or her basic thinking about the issues at stake transparent to the patient (Brody 1989). Patients often want and deserve to know the answer to the question, "What will you do when you find out about my abortion, homosexuality, religious beliefs, moral failures, etc.?" Of course, many patients want to know more than the therapist feels comfortable in sharing. With respect to issues of worldview, the therapist, together with the patient, should try to answer the following basic question: "If I explore further your spiritual concerns (or tell you my own religious identification, join you in a prayer, or suggest a church for you to try), how will this approach help with our work of getting you better?" Without clarity about the patient's thinking on this basic question, it will be difficult for the therapist to affirm that true informed consent has been achieved for treatment of the patient's problems in living.

Summary

Patients' and clinicians' worldviews inevitably shape their attitudes toward clinical problems related to larger human concerns, including identity, hope, meaning and purpose, morality, and autonomy in relation to ultimate authority. Dealing directly with these belief systems in the role of a therapist requires, in addition to assessment of the patient's beliefs, that the therapist be sensitive to the implications of his or her own beliefs and be transparent about his or her aims. The following chapters explore the practical challenges and opportunities of working within several of the world's major frameworks for approaching life.

References

Abernethy AD, Lancia JJ: Religion and the psychotherapeutic relationship: transferential and countertransferential dimensions. J Psychother Pract Res 7:281–289, 1998

American Psychiatric Association: Guidelines regarding possible conflict between psychiatrists' religious commitments and psychiatric practice. Am J Psychiatry 147:542, 1990

American Psychiatric Association: Diagnostic and Statistical Manual of Mental Disorders, 4th Edition, Text Revision. Washington, DC, American Psychiatric Association, 2000

Benson HB: Timeless Healing: The Power and Biology of Belief. New York, Simon & Shuster, 1996

Bilu Y, Witztum E: Working with Jewish Ultra-Orthodox patients: guidelines for a culturally sensitive therapy. Cult Med Psychiatry 17:197–233, 1993

Blackshaw SL, Miller JB: Boundaries in clinical psychiatry (letter). Am J Psychiatry 151:293, 1994

Brody H: Transparency: informed consent in primary care. Hastings Cen Rep 19:5–9, 1989

Commonwealth of Massachusetts: General Guidelines Related to the Maintenance of Boundaries in the Practice of Psychotherapy by Physicians (Adult Patients) (Policy 94-001). Boston, MA, Board of Registration in Medicine, Jan 12, 1994

Frank J: Persuasion and Healing: A Comparative Study of Psychotherapy. Baltimore, MD, Johns Hopkins University Press, 1991

Galanter M, Larson D, Rubenstone E: Christian psychiatry: the impact of evangelical belief on clinical practice. Am J Psychiatry 148:90–95, 1991

Gutheil TG, Gabbard GO: The concept of boundaries in clinical practice: theoretical and risk-management dimensions. Am J Psychiatry 150:188–196, 1993

Gutheil TG, Gabbard GO: Misuses and misunderstandings of boundary theory in clinical and regulatory settings. Am J Psychiatry 155:409–414, 1998

Haldeman DC: Spirituality and religion in the lives of lesbians and gay men, in Textbook of Homosexuality and Mental Health. Edited by Cabaj RP, Stein TS. Washington, DC, American Psychiatric Press, 1996, pp 881–896

Herman JL: Trauma and Recovery. New York, Basic Books, 1992

Horowitz MJ (ed): Person Schemas and Maladaptive Interpersonal Patterns. Chicago, IL, University of Chicago Press, 1991

Kelly TA, Strupp HH: Patient and therapist values in psychotherapy: perceived changes, assimilation, similarity, and outcome. J Consult Clin Psychol 60:34–40, 1992

Kluft RP: Paradigm exhaustion and paradigm shift—thinking through the therapeutic impasse. Psychiatr Ann 22:502–508, 1992

Koenig HG (ed): Handbook of Religion and Mental Health. San Diego, CA, Academic Press, 1998

Meier DE, Emmons CA, Wallenstein S, et al: A national survey of physician assisted suicide and euthanasia in the United States. New Engl J Med 338:1193–1201, 1998

Peteet JR: Approaching spiritual problems in psychotherapy: a conceptual framework. J Psychother Pract Res 3:237–245, 1994

Peteet JR: Putting suffering into perspective: implications of the patient's worldview. J Psychother Pract Res 10:187–192, 2001

Portenoy RK, Coyle N, Kask KM, et al: Determinants of the willingness to endorse assisted suicide: a survey of physicians, nurses, and social workers. Psychosomatics 38:277–287, 1997

Propst LR, Ostrom R, Watkins P, et al: Comparative efficacy of religious and nonreligious cognitive-behavioral therapy for the treatment of clinical depression in religious individuals. J Consult Clin Psychol 60:94–103, 1992

Rational-Emotive Behavior Therapy (REBT). Available at: http://www.rebt.org. Accessed May 15, 2004.

Richards PS, Bergin AE: A Spiritual Strategy for Counseling and Psychotherapy. Washington, DC, American Psychological Association, 1997

Richards PS, Bergin AE: Religious diversity and psychotherapy: conclusions, recommendations, and future directions, in Handbook of Psychotherapy and Religious Diversity. Edited by Richards PS, Bergin AE. Washington, DC, American Psychological Association, 2000, pp 469–489

Schafer R: The psychoanalytic vision of reality. Int J Psychoanal 51:279–298, 1970

Smart Recovery. Available at: http://www.smartrecovery.org. Accessed May 15, 2004.

Wright JH, Beck AT, Thase ME: Cognitive therapy, in The American Psychiatric Publishing Textbook of Clinical Psychiatry, 4th Edition. Edited by Hales RE, Yudofsky SC. Washington, DC, American Psychiatric Publishing, 2003, pp 1245–1284

Yalom ID: Existential Psychotherapy. New York, Basic Books, 1980

PART III

Patients and Their Traditions

CHAPTER 5

Protestant Christians

Mark E. Servis, M.D.

Introduction

Protestant beliefs encompass a wide range of differing traditions and denominations, including Lutheran, Presbyterian, Episcopal or Anglican, Methodist, Evangelical, Fundamentalist, and Pentecostal. Many churches are defined as "Protestant" because they are "not Catholic." While there is a bewildering array of denominations, each with its own specific statements of faith or belief, the differences between them are mostly matters of style and emphasis concerning the nature of religious experience, the degree of reliance on the Bible and church tradition, adherence to specific religious practices, and the nature of communal worship. They all share a commitment to the "good news of the gospel," a message of reconciliation and restoration based on the life and teaching of Jesus Christ.

The mainline Protestant traditions (Lutheran, Presbyterian, and Episcopal) trace their origins to the Protestant Reformation in Europe at the beginning of the sixteenth century. Martin Luther, Ulrich Zwingli, and John Calvin figure prominently in the origins of these mainline Protestant churches. Methodist tradition began with John Wesley, a reformer who intended to bring renewal to the Anglican Church in England. Evangelical and Fundamentalist traditions trace their origins to the model of the New Testament Christian community and later to the Anabaptist traditions originating in Europe around the time of the Reformation. Modern Evangelical and Fundamentalist churches emerged from revival movements in Great Britain and America in the nineteenth century. Both Evangelicals and Fundamentalists are "born-again" Christians who emphasize converting unbelievers to faith, but the Fundamentalists have embraced a more separatist tradition, distancing themselves from secular mainstream culture in the United States. The Pentecostal tradition is an even more recent movement, with most of its development occurring in the United States in the early twentieth century. Pentecostals place an emphasis on the charismatic work of the Holy Spirit and the baptism of the Holy Spirit in believers, as evidenced by "speaking in tongues."

Core Beliefs and Practices

Protestants believe the Bible to be an infallible and authoritative source of truth, to be "God's Word." Protestants believe in one God with three persons (the Trinity)—Father, Son (Jesus Christ), and Holy Spirit. Humanity is separated from God because of its disobedience, which began with Adam and Eve's actions in the Garden of Eden. Although the created world was good, this disobedience led to separation from God and existence in a world filled with suffering, pain, and death. Because of this original sin, humanity now inherits a sinful nature. Sin is any lack of conformity, active or passive, to the moral will of God. Sin may be a matter of action, of thought, or of inner disposition or state. It is the root cause of alienation from God and figures prominently in Protestant thinking and practice. Ongoing acts of disobedience and sin lead to guilt, one way that God tells Protestants that they are "missing the mark." Guilt acts as a signal that reminds Protestants of the need to correct wrong actions and to bring their actions into alignment with God in order to restore a right relationship with Him. But in Protestant theology such "right actions" or good works are insufficient to restore a relationship with a perfect God.

Fortunately God offers a way back to a restored relationship through forgiveness and the needed reparation for sin, something Protestants refer to as "atonement." This atonement occurs through the sacrificial death of Jesus Christ, the Son of God, who was both fully human and fully divine in nature. The redemptive act of Jesus Christ's death on the cross and his resurrection provides a sacrifice through which Protestants can be "saved" from eternal separation from God. This salvation comes from a personal act of faith—recognition of the need for salvation and a willingness to turn to God through belief in Jesus Christ. No other individual, religious practice, or institution is needed for the Protestant to be saved. This idea was at the core of the development of Protestant theology during the Reformation.

The cycle of reform and renewal first evidenced in the Reformation has been an ongoing theme in Protestant tradition, contributing to the bewildering array of denominations and the independence of thought and autonomy of action seen in many churches. Protestant belief is a very individual faith that emphasizes each person's own personal relationship with God and limited concern for the traditions of the church. A broad range of personal interpretation of one's experience of God and of passages from the Bible is permitted, and there is a constant search for the true meaning and interpretation of the scriptures. The more conservative branches of Protestant tradition (Evangelical, Fundamentalist, and Pentecostal) view the mainstream Protestant traditions with some suspicion because of their emphasis on a "social gospel" and their perceived neglect of the message of personal salvation (Thurston 2000). The more mainstream and liberal Protestant churches (Lutheran, Presbyterian, Episcopal or Anglican, Methodist) view sin as embedded in the structures of society and the redemptive message of the gospel as applying not only to individuals but to the culture as a whole (McCullough 2000). These tensions have fueled an ongoing cycle of renewal and reform in Protestant churches that is itself characteristic of the evangelical process.

Clinical Implications

Protestants view all suffering and disease as a consequence of original sin or "the fall" of Adam and Eve in the Garden of Eden as recorded in Genesis in the Bible. Although original sin is the root cause of suffering because it allowed disease and death into the created world, Protestants have differing beliefs regarding sin in the individual and its relationship to an individual's suffering. The idea that an individual's psychiatric disease is a result of personal sin is a common belief among Fundamentalist, Pentecostal, and some Evangelical Protestants, but this belief would not be shared by more mainstream Protestant traditions (Thurston 2000). However, nearly all Protestants would view personal sin, lack of faith, or a spiritual problem as contributing to feelings of depression or anxiety.

Fundamentalist and Pentecostal Protestants sometimes view suffering as a punishment from God for personal sin. They may interpret a specific aspect or time of suffering as being directed or permitted by God because of their own disobedience or sinful action. The idea that God directly influences and controls the events and experiences around the individual Protestant believer to some good purpose is a commonly held perception among Protestants. Protestant patients see sin as having behavioral consequences and view all behaviors as having meaning in the context of their relationship to God. Clinicians need to recognize that, for Protestant patients, sin and suffering have a very complex meaning and significance because they are a reflection of God's work in their life.

Although Protestants will often view sin as contributing to psychiatric illness, they may also see psychiatric illnesses as causing sinful behavior. Psychiatric disorders whose symptoms result in sinful action (sexual promiscuity, paraphilias, lying) or sinful states (pride, arrogance, lust) are clearly in violation of Protestant beliefs regarding Christian conduct. The Protestant patient may be preoccupied with the sinful behaviors associated with his or her psychiatric illness. Protestant patients can also misperceive as sin some behaviors that are part of psychiatric illness, such as obsessions and compulsions.

Protestant beliefs are sometimes used to support ongoing psychopathology or may contribute to the development of psychiatric illness. God is often perceived as overly harsh and punitive, and these perceptions may generate feelings of anxiety, guilt, and anger. Many Protestants fall into a pattern of trying to win God's approval through "right" actions in an attempt to conduct a sinless life. Protestant faith clearly teaches that such legalism ignores and dishonors the atonement of Jesus Christ, a redemption that effectively frees the believer from adherence to an elaborate set of rules. Protestants who are obsessively intent on following rules are trying to make themselves acceptable through what they do and are denying the grace of God. Martin Luther, catalyst of the Protestant Reformation, advanced this doctrine of justification by faith and not works as the centerpiece of Protestant theology. The Protestant believer is not to be a slave to "the law" or driven by guilt, but "free in Christ." The "law" acts as a custodian in bringing the individual to a saving faith in Christ.

Despite these clear theological tenets of Protestant faith, many Protestants present as preoccupied with managing sinful thoughts and behaviors. There can be a legalistic preoccupation with rules and regulations in an attempt to conduct a sinless life. For example, Eric Fromm suggested that the goals of Christian faith were powerlessness and obedience, resulting in a prevailing mood of sorrow and guilt (Fromm 2000). Albert Ellis observed excessive guilt in his devout Christian patients and concluded that the concept of sin promoted psychopathology (Ellis 1971). Distortions or narrow interpretations of Protestant belief can lead to asceticism, legalism, and excessive guilt reactions. But balanced Protestant belief recognizes that such "sin management" techniques are doomed to failure and are rendered unnecessary by the redemption provided through faith in Jesus Christ. Healthy Protestants maintain an awareness of their sinful nature and properly view themselves as part of a universal community that is subject to sin. They see sin as something that affects all people and interferes constantly with the capacity to make good choices, but they do not succumb to excessive self-condemnation and guilt (Carter 1994). The proper response to sin is not to sink further into self-absorption and self-abasement but to recognize a need for a healing relationship with God.

Guilt, like sin, is something that the Protestant patient should recognize but not indulge in excessively. Guilt is seen as a signal that reminds the Protestant of his or her state of original sin and alienation from God. But a continual state of sin is antithetical to Protestant theology. God has forgiven the Protestant of all sin through Jesus Christ's atonement for past, present, and future sin. Through the act of confession and the extension of forgiveness to others, the Protestant enacts the restorative process that God has already bestowed. The Protestant is free from guilt and stands blameless before God. Protestant patients with excessive guilt and self-hate also conflict with Protestant beliefs that affirm the self-worth of the individual, who is made in the image of God (Zackrison 1992).

The following case vignette is an example of a Protestant patient's struggle with excessive and inappropriate guilt:

> Mr. C. was sexually and emotionally abused by his parents during his childhood years. During adolescence he withdrew from his parents, began using drugs heavily, and was sexually irresponsible and promiscuous. In his mid-20s he returned to college, became a Protestant Christian through a campus ministry group, finished an undergraduate degree, and started working. His Protestant conversion was a central organizing element in his sobriety and his new lifestyle. He has been unsuccessful, however, in maintaining steady employment and a healthy marriage due to chronic feelings of guilt, emptiness, and depression. Mr. C.'s devout Protestant belief and history of abuse has led to excessive shame about his past and his lingering feelings of bitterness toward his parents. His ongoing guilt for his continuing failure to live a more successful "Christian" life has contributed to his depression. Mr. C. needs treatment for his depression and associated symptoms, but he also needs to better understand God's gracious redemption, which would free him from personal guilt and shame and allow him to forgive his parents.

Guilt can be excessive and inappropriate in the Protestant patient due to legalistic and harsh interpretations of Protestant belief, but it can also be a healthy signal of the dangerous and destructive effects of sin in his or her life. Guilt is often the trigger that alerts the Protestant patient of the need to take action and even to seek help or treatment.

Another distortion of Protestant belief that may contribute to psychopathology is the perception that the body and particularly sexual drives and behavior are sinful and evil. Men frequently experience guilt over masturbation, an interest in pornography, and sexual behavior outside of marriage. Women have difficulty with sexual repression and inhibition, which may lead to constricted sexual fulfillment in relationships. Although the Bible teaches that the body is a gift from God, Protestants continue to be influenced by Gnostic thinking (a heretical theology in the early Christian church that taught that the body was evil) that true spirituality means neglecting the body to elevate the soul. The result can be an excessively restrictive taboo on all things physical, including the healthy sexual expression that is to be celebrated in Protestant marriage relationships. An example of guilt, depression, and sexual arousal disorder stemming from this distortion of Protestant belief can be found in the following case vignette:

> Ms. S., a devout Protestant, was seen for depression and anxiety related to physical intimacy and sexual conflict in her marriage. She described being motivated to be sexually intimate with her husband; however, during sexual engagement she became flooded with anxiety and recoiled from further contact. In other instances she reported dissociative experiences during sexual relations. Ms. S. believed sexuality was not to be discussed and that sexual fantasy was sinful. Her dilemma was compounded by her Protestant belief that she needed to be submissive to her husband's authority, even in the bedroom. Ms. S.'s distorted Protestant beliefs contributed to the genesis and maintenance of her ongoing psychological conflict around sexuality.

Protestant tradition does put significant restrictions on sexual behavior, which it confines to the context of the committed marriage relationship, but within that setting affirms a full and healthy expression of sexuality.

Some Protestant patients are victims of an exaggerated Protestant work ethic that combines legalism that promotes salvation through "works" or behavior pleasing to God with Jesus' admonition, "Be perfect, therefore, as your heavenly Father is perfect" (New International Version Bible 1985, Matthew 5:48). The pursuit of perfectionism however, can lead to depression and even suicidal ideation and often is supported by an underlying narcissism or obsessive-compulsive personality:

> Mr. V., a young man who recently converted to Protestant belief through a college ministry group, embraced his new faith with enthusiasm and vigor. He began to scrutinize and catalog his sinful behaviors and apply biblical injunctions and strategies to deal with his shortcomings and failures. His life became rigid, stilted, and devoid of pleasurable activities and feelings that distracted him from his goal of perfectionism. When challenged, he would quote a Bible verse, such as, "I can do everything through Christ who gives me strength" (New International Version Bible 1985, Philippians 4:13). After several months of striving and repeated failure to maintain a perfect life, Mr. V. became severely depressed. His narrow and distorted view of how to please God, which was focused on his own efforts and disowning of any personal limitations, was at odds with the Protestant belief that salvation comes through faith and through God's activity, including His work in the lives of believers.

Sometimes Protestant patients may embrace a perfectionist work ethic and not suffer an internal dissonance, but this approach comes at the cost of splitting oneself off from negative feelings. The perfectionist Protestant is not allowed to acknowledge anger toward God, pain, disappointment, or doubt. Unfortunately, this perfectionism also results in a poor ability to tolerate negative feelings in others and promotes attitudes that are dogmatic and legalistic.

Protestant patients may at times present experiences and behavior rooted in their religious beliefs that can be misperceived as evidence of psychopathology by clinicians unfamiliar with Protestant traditions. The diversity of Protestant traditions and the emphasis on the individual interpretation of scripture can create diagnostic challenges. Pentecostals, Fundamentalists, and many Evangelicals speak of the work of God in their lives with an acceptance of supernatural experiences as everyday occurrences. They may confidently report that the voice or action of God in their lives is leading them to insight or truth. Protestants can "hear God's voice" in a moment of crisis or when seeking guidance or direction pertaining to God's will. God sometimes directs seemingly chance events to provide clues or signposts to the Protestant believer, for example, by leading the Protestant to a passage in the Bible or to a particular speaker or pastor who provides a message with special significance to the individual (Thurston 2000). For Protestants, God is engaged in each individual's life, and the believer is expected to have a personal relationship with God that includes God's active involvement in daily and even seemingly mundane affairs. When in doubt about the possibility of psychopathology masquerading as religious belief, clinicians should seek outside help. Individual Protestant beliefs and their interpretation are best benchmarked against the beliefs of fellow Protestants or Protestant clergy in the individual's church.

The Pentecostal "baptism of the Holy Spirit" or "speaking in tongues" is another example of unusual or unique behavior that may appear as psychopathology to the clinician (Dobbins 2000). This excited state of spiritual rapture is evidence of the work of the Holy Spirit in the life of the believer. The resulting unintelligible word salad is usually interpreted by a fellow believer who can relay its significance to the church. To a clinician who has not previously witnessed this ecstatic utterance, glossolalia can look like a flight of ideas reflective of a severe thought disorder, but speaking in tongues is almost always restricted to communal church settings. A second Pentecostal tradition that may be difficult to interpret is the belief in divine healing. Pentecostals believe that prayer for the sick and miracles of healing should be as prominent in the current era as they were in the first-century Church as recorded in the scriptures. Healing comes to the sick through prayer, the laying on of hands, and anointing with oil. The Pentecostal Church has a tradition of gifted "healers" whom God has used to bestow miraculous healing. Pentecostals embrace healing through modern medicine as well, but they are likely to seek divine intervention concurrently (Dobbins 2000).

Several Protestant traditions are both protective and therapeutic for psychiatric illness. The Protestant emphasis on sin and the resulting prohibitions on potentially harmful and unhealthy behaviors promote good medical and psychiatric health. These prohibitions address sexual practices outside of marriage (including premarital sex and marital infidelity), alcohol and drug use, smoking, suicide, and violence. Protestants believe the human body is the "temple of the Holy Spirit" and should be maintained in a healthy state. Consequently Protestants have generally negative views on obesity and tend to promote an active and healthy lifestyle.

Protestants also benefit from their inclination to form very tightly knit communities with a high value placed on mutual support, encouragement, and assistance to those in need. These communities or "fellowships" are usually within individual churches and provide a readily available sense of connectedness to others who share common creeds, standards, and traditions. The Protestant can find compassion, empathy, and a commitment to caring within the fellowship of the church. The more separatist tradition seen in Fundamentalists may create a separate "Christian culture" within the mainstream culture that insulates the believer from the outside world (Thurston 2000).

Many Protestant beliefs and sacred practices are associated with good mental health. Protestant theology emphasizes grace and forgiveness, and many Protestants will be prone to grant forgiveness when they have been hurt by others and are more likely to seek forgiveness when they have wronged others. Prayer, meditation, reading of scripture, fellowship, love and compassion for others, and confession are all practices that are promoted by Protestant traditions and can have direct mental health benefits. Belief in a caring, compassionate, and personal God is a profoundly positive aspect of faith for Protestants. For Protestants, the answers to life's existential questions of meaning, death, existence, and suffering have been addressed and are taught to the believer (McMinn 1996, Post et al. 2000). These spiritual beliefs provide a framework for life that has proved resilient and inspirational to many in the most challenging life circumstances.

Protestant prohibitions on sinful behavior do include some challenging views on controversial aspects of sexuality, morality, and relationships. Protestants largely oppose homosexual behavior as unnatural and contrary to Biblical teaching, although the debate in more liberal mainstream Protestant groups has been active and is evolving toward greater tolerance. This opposition leaves Protestant homosexuals in a difficult bind regarding their relationship with God and within the church. They can choose to pursue a celibate lifestyle with all of its resultant tension and vulnerability to guilt related to sexual urges, or they may seek "deliverance" from homosexuality through religiously mediated change (Davies 2001) or "reparative therapy."

Reparative therapy has been viewed with suspicion by the psychiatric profession as yet another manifestation of homophobia in the culture. Use of reparative therapy remains controversial (Spitzer 2003). Nevertheless, some Protestant churches cautiously endorse such treatment for their homosexual believers. Not surprisingly, homosexual Protestants often suffer from anxiety and depressive disorders in dealing with their underlying sexual orientation. The importance and value of their religious beliefs need to be carefully considered by the clinician in addressing this problem. A quick rejection of foundational religious beliefs central to identity and well-being may not be the answer to the homosexual Protestant's problems. More liberal mainstream Protestant churches are providing more supportive environments based on new, emerging interpretations of the scriptural prohibitions against homosexuality (McCullough et al. 2000).

Protestants view sexual intercourse as the highest form of human intimacy and an experience to be celebrated in marriage only. Sexual practices of all kinds outside of marriage are viewed as sinful. There are differing views on divorce and remarriage, although generally both are discouraged. Most Protestants allow divorce and remarriage in cases of infidelity and abuse. As demographics have shifted, Protestant traditions have become more accepting of divorce, single-parent families, and remarriage. In more conservative Protestant groups, the wife is to "submit" to the authority of the husband (Weaver and Larson 2001). The role of women in the conservative Protestant church is also restricted to more supportive roles, with limited opportunities for leadership. Women's leadership has also been an area of active debate in the Protestant church; broader perspectives on this issue are being considered, and there are new, emerging interpretations of the relevant scriptural passages.

Protestant groups oppose abortion with few exceptions, and the more conservative Fundamentalist, Pentecostal, and Evangelical traditions often support activist roles in opposing abortion in society. Protestants oppose any treatment of children that could be classified as physical or emotional abuse; however, most conservative Protestants accept nonabusive corporal punishment of young children (Goldzband 2000). Children are raised with clear standards of behavior and are expected to submit to and obey parents and authority figures. Alcohol and drug use is vigorously opposed, and more conservative Protestants promote abstinence. Tobacco use is discouraged. Children are not automatically considered to be believers despite being born into Protestant households. They must make a personal decision to be "born again," often in their adolescent years, to establish their own restored relationship with God. As the result of this decision, the Protestant has the assurance of eternal life in heaven with God, which provides hope for a better existence outside this world in the face of suffering and impending death.

Consequently the Protestant believer can claim the biblical truth that "Death has been swallowed up in victory" (New International Version Bible 1985, I Corinthians 15:55).

Variations of Therapeutic Encounters

Protestants have a wide spectrum of attitudes towards mental health and mental health treatment. Adherents to the most conservative Protestant traditions, primarily some Fundamentalists and Pentecostals, have difficulty divorcing mental health from spiritual health. Psychiatric illness is a symptom of a spiritual problem rooted in the believer's relationship with God, and it must be addressed through faithfulness to the Bible and obedience to God's instructions. Only a pastor or a Christian counselor is able to address the spiritual problem that is manifested as psychiatric illness. Prayer, Bible reading, and instruction are the primary treatment modalities. Non-Christian clinicians are viewed with suspicion, unless the problem is clearly "physical" in origin. The work of Jay Adams, a proponent of biblically based Christian counseling, is representative of this approach. His books, *Competent to Counsel* and *More Than Redemption: A Theology of Christian Counseling*, clearly delineate the biblical criteria for mental health and how to achieve it (Adams 1970, Adams 1986, Malony 1998).

More mainstream and liberal Protestant beliefs see mental health as embedded in a broad concept of spiritual health or as somewhat separate and distinct from personal spiritual health. Their conception of spiritual health encompasses personal obedience to biblical teachings, including those focused on creation, justice, and peace. The individual's mental health is best addressed in concert with spiritual health issues, as some degree of interaction and effect is often expected (Malony 1998). Ideally, the clinician would share the Protestant patient's spiritual perspective, although at times this common background may not be necessary because of the limited overlap between mental and spiritual health issues. Most mainstream Protestant patients would put the general skill and competence of the clinician first, with shared religious perspective a close second. A respect for and sensitivity to the mainstream Protestant patient's beliefs and their role in the patient's life is always desired.

Protestants harbor several concerns that sometimes interfere with their access to and use of mental health treatment. A common fear is one of embarrassment in front of fellow believers. This concern is especially found in more conservative Protestant groups that view mental illness as a manifestation of spiritual problems. Many Protestants view anxiety and depression as problems the individual, family, or church should be able to solve. Another concern is that mental health treatment, especially therapy with a non-Christian, will erode or shatter the patient's core religious beliefs. This somewhat paranoid stance can be seen in the antiscience views observed in some conservative Protestant groups that oppose evolution and psychoanalytic theory with equal zeal. Protestant patients may fear that their religious beliefs will be criticized and belittled, the darker sides of their nature exposed, and their faith in God eroded (Malony 1998).

Given these fears and the concerns held by many Protestants who seek mental health treatment, it is important for the clinician to build trust and credibility in the relationship with Protestant patients. For clinicians who share the same Protestant worldview as the patient, there is an opportunity to address spiritual issues that may be embedded in the mental health issues. The Protestant patient will generally respond favorably to the disclosure that the clinician shares the same worldview, and this disclosure will increase trust and improve the therapeutic alliance between the clinician and the patient. Some Protestant patients may expect and even request that spiritual issues be directly addressed in treatment, including the use of religious practices such as prayer and scriptural reading in the treatment sessions. Depending on the nature of the treatment, the necessity for the clinician to remain neutral, and the nature of the patient's problem, religious practices in treatment may indeed be helpful. The Protestant clinician who shares the Protestant patient's worldview needs to be cautious in not overstepping his or her expertise in spiritual matters and should refer the patient to Protestant clergy when appropriate for consultation or adjunctive pastoral counseling.

For the clinician whose worldview differs from that of the Protestant patient, there may be greater challenges in building an effective clinician–patient relationship that can effectively address spiritual and mental health issues. The clinician needs to be able to empathically connect to the patient's worldview and perspective. One suggestion is to use the patient's language, such as "tell me about when you were saved," in exploring his or her frame of reference. It is also essential that the clinician listen to the patient sensitively and from a nonjudgmental perspective. The clinician should be cautious in criticism of the patient's religious perspective, even when the patient expresses doubt or misgivings. The patient's feelings should be validated, but the patient may remain intensely loyal to his or her Protestant beliefs and may simply need a forum to explore ambivalent feelings prohibited in the church setting. The clinician with a different worldview should be quick to consult with Protestant clergy or counselors for advice and input regarding spiritual issues in the treatment and should provide appropriate referral to such help when appropriate.

Collaboration With Faith Communities

The Protestant Church is a valuable resource for Protestant patients, given the recent growth in church-based counseling, especially in the mainstream Protestant denominations. Pastoral counseling services are offered by most churches, and many churches offer counseling and psychotherapy, consultation, and education to church members and sometimes the greater community. Protestant seminaries and schools are increasingly offering graduate-level education in counseling and psychotherapy. Pastors from mainstream Protestant denominations are usually open to collaborating with mental health professionals, and the church is often the first point of contact for Protestants with mental health issues (Post et al. 2000). Clinicians should welcome the opportunity to collaborate with Protestant pastoral counselors, who often have busy caseloads that rival in size those of mental health professionals. One of the most important issues for pastoral counselors is to recognize when to seek the advice of an expert in the mental health field in dealing with a client's psychopathology. Clinicians who offer their consultation services for "tough" cases or who provide education or training for pastoral and lay counselors in the church will develop effective and successful collaborations with clergy who can provide helpful spiritual consultation and assistance in return.

References

Adams JE: Competent to Counsel. Grand Rapids, MI, Baker, 1970

Adams JE: More than Redemption: A Theology of Christian Counseling. Grand Rapids, MI, Baker, 1986

Carter JD: Psychopathology, sin, and the DSM: convergence and divergence. J Psychol Theol 22:277–285, 1994

Davies B: Portraits of Freedom. Downers Grove, IL, InterVarsity Press, 2001

Dobbins RD: Psychotherapy with Pentecostal patients, in Handbook of Psychotherapy and Religious Diversity. Edited by Richards PS, Bergin AE. Washington, DC, American Psychological Association, 2000, pp 155–184

Ellis A: The Case Against Religion: A Psychotherapist's View. New York, Institute for Rational Living, 1971

Fromm E: The Art of Loving. New York, HarperCollins, 2000

Goldzband MG: All God's children: religion, divorce, and child custody. J Am Acad Psychiatry Law 28:408–423, 2000

Malony HN: Religion and mental health from the Protestant perspective, in Handbook of Religion and Mental Health. Edited by Koenig HG. San Diego, CA, Academic Press, 1998, pp 203–211

McCullough ME, Weaver AJ, Larson DB, et al: Psychotherapy with mainline Protestants: Lutheran, Presbyterian, Episcopal/Anglican, and Methodist, in Handbook of Psychotherapy and Religious Diversity. Edited by Richards PS, Bergin AE. Washington, DC, American Psychological Association, 2000, pp 105–130

McMinn MR: Psychology, Theology, and Spirituality in Christian Counseling. Wheaton, IL, Tyndale House, 1996

New International Version Bible. Grand Rapids, MI, Zondervan, 1985

Post SG, Puchalski CM, Larson DB: Physicians and patient spirituality: professional boundaries, competency, and ethics. Ann Intern Med 132:578–583, 2000

Spitzer RL: Can some gay men and lesbians change their sexual orientation? 200 participants reporting a change from homosexual to heterosexual orientation. Arch Sex Behav 32:403–417, 2003

Thurston NS: Psychotherapy with Evangelical and Fundamentalist Protestant patients, in Handbook of Psychotherapy and Religious Diversity. Edited by Richards PS, Bergin AE. Washington, DC, American Psychological Association, 2000, pp 131–154

Weaver AJ, Larson DB: Domestic abuse and religion. Am J Psychiatry 158:822–823, 2001

Zackrison E: A theology of sin, grace, and forgiveness. J Psychol Theol 11:147–159, 1992

CHAPTER 6

Catholic Christians

Judith Moss Hughes, M.D.

Introduction

Since 25% of the population of the United States is Roman Catholic, a working knowledge of the Catholic faith is essential to clinicians' cultural competency. An understanding of Catholicism not only assists the clinician in taking a biopsychosociospiritual history and making a diagnosis, it also helps in formulating plans that integrate the treatment of the whole person.

Christians share with Jews and Muslims a common fatherhood in Abraham, who lived 2,000–3,000 years before Christ. Both Christians and Jews believe scriptural accounts of creation by God, Adam and Eve's fall, and revelations that came through the patriarchs, the prophets, and the Ten Commandments. However, unlike Jews, Christians believe that Jesus Christ is the Messiah, the "Light to the Nations" prophesied by the Old Testament Jewish prophets.

Christians have always considered Jesus to be the Son of God. As the Apostle's Creed states, Jesus "was conceived by the power of the Holy Spirit and born of the Virgin Mary. He suffered under Pontius Pilate, was crucified, died, and was buried. On the third day He rose again. He ascended into heaven and is seated at the right hand of the Father. He will come again to judge the living and the dead" (Catechism of the Catholic Church 1997, nn. 198–1065). Christians believe not only that Jesus' life and teachings reveal what God is like and how humanity is called to live but that His suffering, death, and resurrection reunited humanity with God. This act of love liberated humankind from the grip of sin and death. Jesus offers eternal life to those who believe in Him.

When He was on earth, Jesus chose 12 apostles. He appointed one of the apostles, Peter, to lead the Church (New American Bible 1986, Matthew 16:16–19). Catholics trace the authority of the Pope, who is elected by a council of cardinals (bishops who serve as advisors and administrators), to his succession from Peter, the first Pope. Christians date the birth of the church to the day during the Jewish feast of Pentecost (50 days after Christ's resurrection and 10 days after Christ's ascension into heaven) when the Holy Spirit came to the apostles and Jesus' mother, Mary, in Jerusalem. The Bible records that the Holy Spirit came in the form of a wind and small fires that rested above their heads and empowered them to speak in many languages. Thousands who witnessed this event and heard Peter preach became followers of Jesus. As people have since that time, they became Christians by receiving the Spirit of Christ in the sacred ritual of baptism. Saint Ignatius of Antioch first used the term Catholic Church when he wrote around 107 A.D., "Where there is Jesus Christ, there is the Catholic Church" (Catechism of the Catholic Church 1997, n. 830).

Before leaving this earth, Christ promised His followers that He would always remain with them—when they prayed and healed in His name; when they performed acts of charity, mercy and service; and especially when they gathered to worship God in the eucharistic meal of consecrated bread and wine, which for Catholics is the real presence of Jesus.

As it spread, the Christian faith began to both influence and be influenced by Greek and Roman philosophers. For example, early Church council members who struggled with how to describe Jesus and God borrowed the Latin word *persona* first used by Cicero. The Christian philosopher Boethius (ca. 480–525) later defined a person as "an individual substance with a rational nature" (Boethius 1918, p. 91). This concept, along with other meanings the word had gathered from the Greeks, became the basis of the doctrine of the Trinity: that God is one divine nature possessed equally by three distinct Persons who are distinguished only by their relation to one another, that Jesus is one of the Divine Persons, and that He possesses two distinct natures, one of which is divine and the other human. This Trinitarian concept of God is unique to Christians. Personhood is an attribute shared by God, the angels, and human persons. God and the angels are pure spirits; human persons are embodied spirits. Christians eventually incorporated the philosophy of Aristotle and that of Saint Thomas Aquinas (ca. 1225–1274) into the concept that the human person is an inseparable unity of body and soul—the soul being "the spiritual principle of life" (Catechism of Catholic Church 1997, nn. 363, 365).

After centuries of persecution, Christianity became the established religion of the Roman Empire under Constantine. A number of controversies have since challenged the Church's unity and dominance. In 1054, the Eastern Orthodox and the Roman Catholic Churches divided over disagreements on Trinitarian dogma. In the sixteenth century, Martin Luther initiated another major schism by publicly listing his points for reform that centered on the Catholic doctrines regarding justification, good works and grace, the roles of scripture and tradition, and the practice of selling indulgences. Reform turned into violent protest and many "Protestants" separated from the Catholic Church.

Concurrent with the Protestant Reformation, the philosophy of secular humanism in the European universities strongly weakened theology's influence in academia and caused a falling away from the Catholic understanding of the hierarchical unity of knowledge. For humanists, moral standards became a relativistic matter. Descartes and his followers viewed the human body as an object to be dissected, manipulated, and analyzed, rather than a subject that manifested spiritual personhood. While the Cartesian separation of body and mind allowed the expansion of medical and scientific research, the meaning of "soul" and "mind" continued to change. As freedom was perceived by some as freedom from moral restraints and theological dogma, psychology and psychiatry claimed increasing expertise concerning mind and brain. Interior dialogue with God gave way to an introspective dialogue with the psychological self and the therapist, leaving the soul, morality, and the transcendent in the domain of the church.

The views underlying the revolutionary movements of the eighteenth century continued to position the Church and its moral authority as an enemy to freedom. In disagreement, Catholics see themselves as valuing freedom—freedom being the very medium for seeking and knowing truth, love, and excellence in all endeavors (Pinckaers 1993). Nineteenth-century thinkers, including Charles Darwin, Karl Marx, Friedrich Nietzsche, and Sigmund Freud, dealt further blows to the Catholic concepts of freedom and human dignity. In psychiatry, Freud was viewed suspiciously because of his atheism and writings that viewed Catholicism as regressive and neurotic. In defense of Catholicism, the French Jewish philosopher Henri Bergson, concluded after 25 years of research that the Catholic saints and mystics had exceptional mental health, supreme good sense, intellectual vigor, joy, simplicity, an inclination for action, adaptability, firmness, and spiritual discernment (Bergson 1935).

The American public viewed Catholics as patriotic Americans during World War I and World War II, and the faith enjoyed unprecedented popularity in the United States in the 1950s. However, Pope Paul VI's condemnation of birth control in his 1968 letter *Humanae Vitae* (Pope Paul VI 1968) led to widespread dissension both in Europe and in America. The Second Vatican Council (1962–1965), convened to "open the windows" of the Church to a changing world, produced sweeping changes. The Mass, or liturgy of Word and Eucharist, was no longer said in Latin. Priests turned from the altar to face the people, the altar was moved into more open space, and churches were stripped of kneeling rails and ornate statuary. Catholics could confess while meeting face-to-face with the priest, and they could receive Holy Communion in the hand rather than directly on the tongue. Protestant baptisms were accepted as valid, Protestant hymns appeared in Catholic hymnals, and ecumenical dialogues developed. In the years since the Second Vatican Council, the number of priests and nuns has declined and the role of educated laity has increased.

In his first encyclical letter, Pope John Paul II (1979) envisioned a civilization of life and love. Influential in defeating communism in Poland, Pope John Paul II attempted to confront scandal, dissent, and decay within the Church by uniting the remaining strands of Christian thought in Western culture into a philosophy known as Christian humanism or Christian existential personalism (Weigel 1999). He emphasized the dignity of the human person from conception to natural death in the face of threats such as consumerism and technology and encouraged all persons to work together for the common good (Pope John Paul II 1995). In addition, he asked the Church to "purify its memory" by seeking forgiveness for all the injustices done by Catholic individuals against Jews, Muslims, Protestants, Indians, Africans, women, and other Catholics (Accatolli 1998).

Contemporary Catholics are ethnically, socioeconomically, and politically diverse. One-third of Catholics are between age 18 and 29 years. Worldwide, Hispanics, Asians, and Africans constitute the fastest growing Catholic populations. Differences in how these groups celebrate and live the same faith can be instructive for clinicians. Theologically, Catholics represent a spectrum ranging from liberal to traditional (or Orthodox). Typically, one-third are highly committed to practicing their faith, one-third are moderately committed (attending church one or two times a month), and one-third have little or no contact with church.

Core Beliefs and Practices

The *Catechism of the Catholic Church*, officially approved by the Pope in 1992, has been translated into many languages and is a helpful summary of what the Catholic Church professes and practices (Catechism of the Catholic Church 1997). The first section concerns the creeds, and the second describes the seven sacraments of the Church. The third section covers concepts of practical living, and the fourth discusses prayer. The third section, entitled "Life with Christ," addresses topics of particular interest to clinicians, including the desire for happiness, freedom and responsibility, morality and conscience, sin and the virtues, and social justice.

Catholics share basic creeds or professions of faith with almost all Christians, including the Apostle's Creed and the Nicene Creed (Catechism of the Catholic Church 1997, nn. 26–1065). Similarly, the Ten Commandments (New American Bible 1986, Exodus 20) and the Beatitudes of Jesus (New American Bible 1986, Matthew 5:3–11) are fundamental moral codes that are important to both Protestants and Catholics.

Sacraments are distinctive Church practices that mediate God's grace to people. Catholics believe that Jesus instituted seven sacraments: baptism, penance and reconciliation (previously confession), the Eucharist (Holy Communion), confirmation, marriage, holy orders (ordination to the priesthood and diaconate), and the anointing of the sick (previously extreme unction). Catholics believe that in the centrally important Eucharistic meal, bread and wine when consecrated by the priest become the Real Presence of Christ's Body, Blood, Soul, and Divinity. Accordingly, when Catholics receive the Eucharist, they are receiving Jesus Christ and offering themselves in unity with Him. As members of the Body of Christ, the Church, including believers past and present, act as members of His Mystical Body. Catholics are obliged to attend Mass every Sunday and on holy days of obligation for special religious holidays. Many Catholic churches offer daily Mass, and committed Catholics often participate on a daily basis. The Church recommends confession on a monthly basis and requires confession before reception of the Eucharist if one has committed a grave, or mortal, sin.

Following Christ means loving God and one's neighbor as oneself through performing good works, avoiding sin, bearing one's cross of suffering, and developing virtues so as to love more perfectly (see New American Bible 1986, I Corinthians, Chapter 13 and Matthew 5:3–11). For centuries, the Church has encouraged believers to imitate Christ in performing the "seven corporal acts of mercy" (clothing the naked, feeding the hungry, visiting the imprisoned, giving drink to the thirsty, sheltering the homeless, visiting the sick, and burying the dead) and the "seven spiritual works of mercy" (admonishing the sinner, instructing the ignorant, counseling the doubtful, comforting the sorrowful, bearing wrongs patiently, forgiving injuries, and praying for the living and the dead). Catholic patients who are self-preoccupied and socially isolated can find among these precepts excellent behavioral goals for developing character.

Catholics speak of character in terms of virtue and vice. Virtues are habitual attitudes that shape a healthy mind and soul. In addition to human virtues, such as the cardinal virtues borrowed from ancient Greece (prudence, justice, fortitude, and temperance), Catholics emphasize the theological virtues (faith, hope, and love) that are granted by God. Virtues are opposed by corresponding vices—for example, generosity by greed. To master a particular vice such as lust, a person would need to cultivate appropriate virtues such as chastity, temperance, and continence. Capital vices (envy, pride, lust, covetousness, gluttony, anger, and sloth) engender other vices or sins. Catholics understand sin as "an offense against God and an offense against reason, truth, and right conscience" (Catechism of the Catholic Church 1997, nn. 1849–1850).

Catholics believe that the personal conscience, which is formed and educated in the precepts of the Church, helps the individual both to hear the voice of God and to determine what is just, right, and good. The church teaches that all persons have a free will and the right to act according to their consciences. The choices they make then determine the state they enter after life ends. Catholicism teaches that there are four such states: 1) a state for children who die without baptism (sometimes referred to as limbo); 2) purgatory, the state of final purification before entrance into heaven; 3) heaven, the state of supreme happiness of eternal life with God and the blessed; and 4) hell, the state of self-exclusion from communion with God, reserved for those who refuse by their own free will to believe and to be converted from sin.

Catholics consider human life from conception to natural death to be sacred, since the Holy Bible states that humans were created in the image of God. Since God is Spirit and Love, the person is always viewed in the context of relationships with others in the family, workplace, community, and Church. For Catholics, contraception, sterilization, in vitro fertilization, and embryonic stem cell cloning offend this relationship with God; the first two separate life from love, and the last two separate love from life. Catholics regard abortion as homicide because it is a refusal of both life and love. Because marriage is a sacramental covenant between a man and a woman for life, divorce is not recognized. Catholics can annul marriage vows only if they did not freely choose to marry because of external influences (e.g., an arranged marriage) or internal influences (e.g., deception, drugs, or irrational thinking). Natural family planning, or abstinence from intercourse during the woman's fertile days, is the only permissible means of spacing births.

Catholics also draw practical implications at the end of life from their view that the person is a steward of the body, not its owner. Since believers should give reasonable care and attention to one's body but not seek life at any cost, a terminally ill person may refuse treatment that is disproportionate in burden to any benefits. They should not, however, refuse or be refused food and water, as they are not treatments, but necessary requirements for life. While taking one's own or another person's life is wrong, the Church recognizes that the mind of the suicidal person may have been impaired by psychopathology, and so grants victims of suicide a church funeral and burial, leaving judgment to God.

Catholics believe that suffering and death have been a part of human existence since Adam and Eve sinned. However, they believe that Jesus' death gave suffering redemptive meaning and that following Christ (taking up one's own "cross" for the love of Christ) can bring benefits. Pope John Paul II (1984) in his apostolic letter, "On the Christian Meaning of Human Suffering," discusses several of those benefits: 1) the unleashing of love in the human person so that acts of love are performed for others; 2) the completion of what is lacking in Christ's afflictions for the sake of the Church; 3) a call or vocation to the virtues of perseverance, fortitude, and courage; 4) a drawing closer to Christ in the sharing of His cross; 5) a path for religious conversion; 6) the gaining of spiritual maturity for the sufferer; and 7) a call to the transcendent, or going beyond oneself.

Prayer is an essential part of the Christian life because it expresses and shapes the personal relationship between the believer and God. Prayer can take several forms, including singing hymns. Many prayers, such as the Lord's Prayer, the morning offering, grace before and after meals, the liturgy of the hours, and the rosary, have remained the same throughout the ages. Mental or contemplative prayer (as in silent adoration before Christ in the Blessed Sacrament in the tabernacle) is a spontaneous, personal dialogue with God that involves listening receptively. Speaking in tongues, or glossolalia, is a rare type of prayer experienced as a gift of the Holy Spirit by Catholics in the charismatic movement of the church. In prayer, a Catholic can ask forgiveness, make a request on behalf of him- or herself or another person (as in praying for those who are ill), or express thanksgiving and praise. Catholics believe that private and communal prayer can include living and deceased believers (the "communion of saints") who intercede for each other. For example, a Catholic might request intercession to Jesus from a saint in heaven as well as from a living fellow believer. However, Catholics, like all Christians, regard Jesus as the only intercessor and mediator with God the Father on behalf of all humanity. Because Mary is Jesus' mother and recognized by Catholics as their mother, prayers to Mary are centered on the person of Christ (Catechism of the Catholic Church 1997, nn. 2673–2679). Fasting and almsgiving often accompany prayer, especially during the liturgical season of Lent. When fasting is an ascetical practice of self-denial that expresses penance, it should not be confused with an eating disorder.

Clinical Implications

In taking an initial history, a clinician may need to explain the reason for asking about the patient's faith. The spiritual history contains important information about the meaning that religious affiliation brings to the patient's experiences. A complete religious, spiritual, or moral history of a Catholic patient should include the following elements: 1) a faith history of how the patient became Catholic, whether he or she is currently a practicing Catholic, and, if not, why; 2) a sacramental history that includes age at baptism and confirmation and the frequency of penance and Eucharist; 3) a family faith history of the religions of the patient's mother, father, spouse, and children; 4) a brief prayer history, including types and frequency of prayer; 5) a history of involvement in parish activities, church ministries, and volunteer programs; 6) a statement regarding personal goals in life, sources of greatest happiness, and perception of life after death; and 7) a review of areas related to morality in general (a "moral history").

Taking a moral history will help the clinician ascertain whether the patient could benefit from a spiritual consultation with a priest, pastoral counselor, or spiritual director. Examples of patients who could benefit from a spiritual consultation include Catholic patients with depression and anxiety related to adultery, divorce and remarriage, abortion, pornography, gambling, addiction, and domestic violence or other forms of abusive behavior. Unlike a priest who asks a person to list sins during confession, a clinician who is taking a moral history will ask more general questions; for example, Are you struggling with a past or present sense of moral failure or weakness at this time? How does this sense relate to your current conflicts? What aspects of your religion have you found helpful during this time? Have you talked with a priest or spiritual director about such problems in the past? Does this person know of your decision to seek medical attention or psychotherapy? Would you be interested in discussing the moral and religious aspects of your problems with a priest?

When they are ill, Catholics often seek the prayers of their pastor and parish, and the request may be publicly announced in the context of a religious service. They can also request that a priest conduct the sacrament of the anointing of the sick. Patients with psychiatric conditions tend to be offered more privacy, as priests regard patient confidentiality as similar to their obligation to keep absolutely secret what has been told to them in the confessional. Moral failures are regarded as matters between God and the sinner, and if parishioners' prayers are requested, the reason for the request is likely to be worded in general terms.

Another reason for taking a moral history is to clarify whether the Catholic patient's presenting symptoms are aggravated or complicated by particular moral transgressions. The clinician may be able to address such a patient's need for particular virtues—for example, for fortitude to master anxiety, perhaps one of the conditions most closely related to spiritual problems. In every Catholic Mass, the priest prays, "Free us from all anxiety." In many of his writings and talks, Pope John Paul II repeatedly states, "Be not afraid!" much as Christ commanded, "Fear not!" The Bible teaches that

"There is no fear in love, but perfect love drives out fear because fear has to do with punishment, and so one who fears is not yet perfect in love" (New American Bible 1986, I John 4:18).

Some Catholics with anxiety feel an additional burden of shame and inadequacy because they understand that the victory of Christ on the cross leaves no reason for human fear. These patients may find helpful the distinctions made by the theologian-philosopher Hans Urs von Balthasar (2000), who distinguished among existential anxiety (that is morally neutral), the anxiety of the wicked (marked by isolation, deception, rigidity, despair, loss of contact with reality, and paranoia), and the anxiety of the good. This latter anxiety is accompanied by humility, earnest concern for others, fear of God and his judgment, and a turning toward God for mercy. Such anxiety in Christians can stem from a fear of suffering, a lack of hope, a troubled conscience, diminishing religious commitment, or a feeling that one is not as faithful as one claims to be. Therefore, like suffering, anxiety can be a call to conversion, repentance, and reconciliation with God.

Catholic patients may present with inappropriately severe feelings of guilt about what could be a sin and with doubts about whether their confessions are complete enough for forgiveness from God. Some of these patients have a condition known as scrupulosity, a religious form of obsessive-compulsive disorder. On the other hand, clinicians may see a religious variant of sociopathy that is marked by an absence of guilt in the presence of serious moral transgression in a person who professes a religious commitment. Consider the example of a middle-aged priest who presents with anxiety symptoms and reports that his girlfriend just had an abortion. His appearance is well groomed, and his mood is pleasant; he reveals no sense of anguish or responsibility for his role in conceiving a child. Instead of engaging in introspection and searching for forgiveness, he insists that he has a "biochemical imbalance" and requests tranquilizers. Such individuals use a superficial religious demeanor to manipulate others for secondary gain.

After conducting the spiritual, religious, and moral history, the clinician identifies problems that could benefit from integration of the patient's life and faith and then formulates a treatment plan that respects the roles and boundaries of all involved. The initial goal of the clinician will be to restore physical functioning—sleep, appetite, and energy—and then the ability of the patient to perceive reality, coordinate judgments, and control excessive emotion. The priest's goal will be to promote the spiritual welfare of the Catholic patient, but both priests and clinicians can encourage even patients with major mental illness to draw on their spirituality for strength and perseverance. The acronym PRIEST summarizes the spiritual expectations of the Catholic patient, which the clinician should understand, as they will affect treatment:

P—The *priest* is responsible for the care of the patient's spiritual soul.

R—*Respect* the teachings and traditions of the Catholic faith.

I—Include the *Interior Life* of conscience, will, prayer, faith, hope, and love.

E—Address the *Exterior Life* of good works, virtues, family, and community.

S—The *Sacramental Life* brings grace, healing, and forgiveness.

T—*Treat* others as you would want them to treat you (Golden Rule).

When a prominent Catholic priest or lay leader is afflicted with alcoholism, pedophilia, or pederasty, experienced mental health professionals may need to collaborate closely (at times in secure settings) with priests, pastoral counselors, or spiritual directors who are familiar with psychiatric disorders. In cases in which bishops and their psychological consultants confuse the criminal and legal, moral and religious, and psychological and neurobiological aspects of the person's behavior, major problems result, as seen in the current crisis in the Catholic Church's management of these problems.

Many patients present with conflicts that involve discord between Catholic teaching and contemporary Western culture. Frequently seen areas of conflict include self-promotion versus self-denial, feelings versus faith and reason, individual autonomy versus the community good, biological versus spiritual explanations for human problems, truth as relative versus truth as absolute, suffering as meaningless versus suffering as redemptive, and sexuality as recreation versus sexuality as interpersonal spousal communion with the potential for creating human life. Examples of patients for whom these conflicts are relevant in clinical care include those who are struggling with homosexual behavior, conjugal intercourse with contraception, premarital and extramarital sexual relations, marriage between persons who have had a civil divorce, and postabortion emotional responses.

"First, do no harm" has been a general guiding principle in medical ethics for centuries. Both Catholic and non-Catholic therapists often find it challenging to avoid influencing patients on the basis of their own personal attitudes and beliefs. For example, a non-Catholic therapist who is treating a patient who was sexually abused by a priest accepts without question the patient's statement that the church is hypocritical and an unreliable guide for living. The therapist reflects later that his own feelings about the misuse of authority had prevented him from exploring the patient's deep ambivalence toward the Catholic faith tradition. He realizes that he has missed an opportunity in assisting the patient to correct a cognitive distortion, and as a result the patient's progress was slowed.

Varieties of Therapeutic Encounters

Clinical encounters involving three types of dyads deserve special mention: a Catholic therapist and Catholic patient, a Catholic therapist and a non-Catholic patient, and a non-Catholic therapist and Catholic patient. Catholic therapists often receive referrals from patients and priests. In some geographical areas, lack of Catholic mental health professionals can be a barrier to treatment for traditional Catholics. However, most Catholics prefer to see a clinician who is a well-trained, respected professional and do not consider religious affiliation alone as a marker for professional competence. For some Catholic patients, including those who are experiencing guilt and associated emotional distress (for example, after an abortion), a Catholic therapist can potentially achieve a stronger therapeutic alliance because the therapist and patient share beliefs regarding sin, conscience, and forgiveness.

A Catholic therapist who is treating a non-Catholic patient can focus on universal values that humanity shares in common. There may be times, however, when a Catholic therapist and non-Catholic patient cannot find morally common ground, as, for example, when the patient expects the therapist to support or facilitate choices to proceed with abortion or assisted suicide. Catholic physicians continue to take seriously the prohibition in the Hippocratic oath against assisting in an abortion. Catholics also maintain that women who are seeking help with a problem pregnancy have a right to be completely informed about all of the risks of abortion, including the physical, psychological, and spiritual risks, and to receive information on all aspects of fetal development and other options besides abortion, including adoption. The Catholic physician or therapist must balance personal conviction with a responsibility to see that the patient is fully informed before making a medical decision with serious moral implications. The compassionate Catholic clinician should take care that a patient who chooses abortion does not feel abandoned, rejected, or condemned, and should always be oriented toward life and not death, toward love and not fear, and toward truth and not deception.

At times Catholic patients will be more comfortable discussing sexual and moral issues with a non-Catholic therapist, because they may feel more at ease in what they perceive to be a nonjudgmental setting. Clearly, patients who have been victims of sexual abuse by a priest may feel unable to discuss their past with a Catholic therapist because of the transference of anger and mistrust. However, non-Catholic clinicians should align with the patient's religious identity in order to form a more comfortable therapeutic alliance. The more knowledgeable the clinician is about Catholic beliefs, practices, and resources, the more he or she will be able to help Catholic patients understand and resolve their difficulties.

Collaboration With Faith Communities

The resources of the Catholic Church are open to all. Clinicians can obtain a diocesan directory of parishes, retreat centers, and human services agencies from the bishop's chancery of the diocese. Most dioceses also provide a listing of approved spiritual directors with whom the mental health clinician can work jointly. Many pastoral counseling centers also have Catholic counselors. Seminarians, priests, and nuns who need mental health care should be treated in coordination with their religious superiors, who usually initiate referrals to sites that specialize in psychotherapy within the Catholic framework. The National Conference of Catholic Bishops, the National Catholic Bioethics Center, and the Catholic Medical Association publish educational materials and directives on all aspects of health care. Many Catholic organizations have Web sites that are listed in the book *Catholics on the Internet*, by Brother John Raymond (2000).

Catholic service agencies have various resources that can support patients with mental disorders and augment clinical care, providing the resources of a supportive community for patients facing homelessness, hunger, domestic violence, and crisis pregnancies, among other problems. One well-known model for collaboration of the church, the community, and clinicians is found in Gheel (Geel), Belgium, where for centuries the Catholic healing shrine, private citizens, and the clinical setting have worked together to care for mentally ill patients. Clinicians would do well to find or perhaps even initiate such services in their own communities (for an example of such services in the United States, see www.spiritofgheel.org).

References

Accattoli L: When a Pope Asks for Forgiveness. Translated by Aumann J. Staten Island, NY, Alba House, 1998

Bergson H: The Two Sources of Morality and Religion. Translated by Audra RA, Brereton C. New York, Henry Holt and Company, 1935

Boethius: The Theological Tractates and the Consolation of Philosophy. Translated by Stewart HF, Rand EK, Tester, SJ. Cambridge, MA, Loeb Classical Library, 1918

Brother John Raymond: Catholics on the Internet. Rocklin, CA, Prima Publishing, 2000

Catechism of the Catholic Church, English translation, 2nd Edition. Washington, DC, US Catholic Conference—Libreria Editrice Vaticana, 1997

New American Bible, Saint Joseph Edition. New York, Catholic Book Publishing Company, 1986

Pinckaers S: The Source of Christian Ethics. Washington, DC, Catholic University Press, 1993

Pope John Paul II: The Redeemer of Man. Boston, MA, Daughters of Saint Paul, 1979

Pope John Paul II: On the Christian Meaning of Human Suffering. Boston, MA, Daughters of Saint Paul, 1984

Pope John Paul II: The Gospel of Life. Boston, MA, Pauline Books and Media, 1995

Pope Paul VI: Human Vitae. Boston, MA, Daughters of Saint Paul, 1968

von Balthasar HU: The Christian and Anxiety. San Francisco, CA, Ignatius Press, 2000

Weigel G: Witness to Hope: The Biography of Pope John Paul II. New York, Harper-Collins, 1999, pp 130–139

CHAPTER 7

Jews

David Greenberg, M.A., M.B., B.Chir., M.R.C.Psych.

Irving S. Wiesner, M.D.

Introduction

The history of the Jewish people is first recorded in the Torah (the first five books of the Old Testament) and the remainder of the Old Testament. Catholicism, Protestantism, and Islam all trace their roots to this common source and to this people. The Bible chronicles the formation of the Jewish nation from Abraham through Isaac, Jacob, and Joseph. Their travel to Egypt during a time of famine and their growth in numbers and subsequent oppression as slaves in that land is followed by their deliverance from bondage through the divinely enacted plagues and the miraculous dividing of the Red Sea. The remainder of the Old Testament describes their victories and defeats and the many lessons they learned.

The Jewish people played a major role in the pages of the New Testament, and Jews were the exclusive members of the earliest Christian Church. The early Christians (Jews and Gentiles [non-Jews]) and the Rabbinical Jews (those who continued to follow the precepts of the Old Testament as interpreted by the rabbis) went their separate ways. The centrality of the Temple and animal sacrifice, which was a vital part of Jewish worship, was no longer possible after the destruction of the Temple in Jerusalem in the year 70 A.D., because the Temple was the only place at which these vital rituals could be performed. Synagogues became the focus of communal worship for the Jewish people after they were scattered among the nations in what is known as the Diaspora. The Jewish leaders (rabbis) who succeeded the judges and prophets of the Old Testament interpreted Holy Scripture and applied its truths to daily living for the guidance of their congregants.

Throughout history most Jews remained true to their identity in many lands and cultures, although they were often oppressed and persecuted. Over the centuries, Jews maintained their culture and religious practices in the closed communities in which they were forced to live. In Europe the social change that occurred during the eighteenth century, in the era known as the Enlightenment, allowed Jews the opportunity to mingle with the outside world. This intermingling in turn led to struggles concerning the maintenance of Jewish identity and the appropriate degree of integration with the larger culture. Some feared assimilation and the eventual disappearance of their unique Jewish mission. Others welcomed, in varying degrees, the opportunity to participate in the wider society with all of its opportunities. From these struggles and choices came the more recent divisions among a people who, despite their differences, strongly cling to a general unity of identity.

Worldwide, Jews number approximately 14 million, a small number compared to other faith groups, such as Christianity with about 1.9 billion, Islam with 1.1 billion, and Hinduism with 780 million (Information Please Almanac 2004). In the United States, the number of Jews is approximately 5.6 million (Ash 1997), greater than the number of Jews in Israel, which is 5.5 million. Although Jews constitute only 2% of the overall United States population, they make up 9.1% of the New York State population and 5.5% of the New Jersey proportion. New York City is the city with the world's largest Jewish population, a total of 1.8 million (Ash 1997).

Core Beliefs and Practices

A 2002 survey of American Jews by the American Jewish Committee pointed out that only 51% reported membership in a synagogue, although 70% identified with a particular branch of Judaism (American Jewish Committee 2003). Although the major subdivisions of Judaism are distinguished by features that will be described subsequently, it is worth noting that 30% of Jews who responded to the 2002 survey did not belong to a synagogue nor did they identify with any particular branch of Judaism.

Reform Judaism "emphasize[s] the Jewish prophetic values and accept[s] Jewish practices that it considers relevant for modern times" (survey criterion from the 1990 National Jewish Population Survey; North American Jewish Data Bank 2001). Reform Jews account for 30% of American Jews who identify with a branch of Judaism (American Jewish Committee 2003). Reform Jews focus on the autonomy of the individual and thus support each person's right to decide how to live out his or her faith tradition. They see themselves differently from more ritually observant Jews because of their belief that their sacred heritage has evolved and adapted over time and should continue to do so (Union of American Hebrew Congregations 2002).

Reconstructionist Jews compose just 2% of American Jews who identify with a branch of Judaism (American Jewish Committee 2003) and "represent a humanistic approach to Jewish tradition that redefines the concept of God in humanistic terms" (North American Jewish Data Bank 2001). Reconstructionist Judaism contrasts itself to Orthodox Judaism in that it "does not view Judaism as a total and immutable revelation from God to Moses at Sinai that is essentially unchanged through all generations... [but rather]...as the ever evolving product of history, an ongoing attempt to forge a society based on holy values" (Jewish Reconstructionist Federation 2000). Reconstructionist Jews further delineate the differences as follows (Jewish Reconstructionist Federation 2000): "Reconstructionism diverges from Conservative Judaism in terms of priorities. We believe that the basic tenets of Judaism need to be re-examined and restated for our age. We see this as a more pressing priority than the particulars of the Jewish law." Finally, "reconstructionism differs from Reform Judaism, however, concerning how much of the tradition needs to be preserved." Reconstructionism emphasizes social reform—on "incorporating contemporary mores into the Jewish experience with regard to the role of women, respect for individual liberties, and acceptance of cultural pluralism." Reconstructionist Jews work actively with international conflict resolution and with hunger, civil rights, and environmental issues.

The Conservative Jew "asserts the continuing authority of Jewish law as part of a dynamic and developing tradition" (North American Jewish Data Bank 2001). About 31% of American Jews who identify with a branch of Judaism are Conservative Jews (American Jewish Committee 2003). It is difficult to encapsulate the beliefs of this religious group, and often their own concepts differ from those ascribed to them by observers outside the group. A statement outlining their position points out that

> Conservative Judaism is best understood as a sacred cluster of core values. No single prepositional statement comes close to identifying its center of gravity. Nor does Conservative Judaism occupy the center of the contemporary religious spectrum because it is an arbitrary and facile composite of what may be found on the left or the right. On the contrary, its location flows from an organic and coherent world view best captured in terms of core values of relatively equal worth (Schorsch 1995).

These core values are 1) the centrality of modern Israel; 2) Hebrew as the irreplaceable language of Jewish expression; 3) devotion to the ideal of *Klal Yisrael* (which refers to the affirmation that all Jews, regardless of their beliefs, are valued and are part of the Jewish people); 4) the defining role of Torah in the reshaping of Judaism; 5) the study of Torah; 6) the governance of Jewish life by *halakha* (the system of Jewish law as interpreted by rabbinical authority); and 7) belief in God (Schorsch 1995).

The Orthodox "emphasize the binding unchanging character of Jewish law" (North American Jewish Data Bank 2001). Seven percent of American Jews who identify with a branch of Judaism are Orthodox Jews (American Jewish Committee 2003). This number includes the Modern Orthodox as well as the Ultra-Orthodox Jews.

Modern Orthodox Jews attempt to bridge the gap between the values of fully observant Judaism and the modern world. They support the truths of Ultra-Orthodox Judaism while interacting more fully with the culture around them. The Modern Orthodox Jewish male will wear Western clothes but will also always wear a hat or a distinctive head covering called a yarmulke or *kippah*. Married women will cover their hair with a scarf or wear a wig for modesty. In general, the Modern Orthodox Jew "maintains the range of religious practices while being an active member of the secular world, accepting any kind of work and study as long as it does not overtly contravene religious law" (Greenberg 2001, p. 570).

Ultra-Orthodox Jews are members of the most theologically conservative form of Judaism, also known as Haredi Judaism. *Haredi* means "fearful of God" (Ultra-Orthodox Judaism 2003) and points to their piety and adherence to what they believe to be the most observant form of belief and practice. They see themselves as the defenders of the faith and consider their belief system and religious practices to follow most closely God's law as given on Mount Sinai. This group accounts for a small portion of the overall Jewish community in the United States (it is relatively larger in Israel), but it has much greater overall significance than its numbers would suggest. Ultra-Orthodox Judaism is seen as the "gold standard" of Judaism by some and as an example of the dangers of isolationism and authoritarianism by others. Ultra-Orthodox Jews are the most difficult of the Jewish subgroups to reach for psychiatric treatment. Some of the unique features of its members and some of the issues involved in their treatment will be the focus of the latter portion of this chapter.

Each subgroup of Judaism has a range of rich and sometimes subtle underlying beliefs and practices, and these features within and among subdivisions frequently overlap. Even among the Ultra-Orthodox, whose members are the most separated from secular society, there are many schools of adherents led by revered rabbis, including Hasidism, Chabad-Lubavich, Neo-Orthodoxy, Religious Zionism, and Messianic Zionism. The dietary laws, observance of the Sabbath, the role of men and women in the worship service as well as the community and in marriage, the use of Hebrew in worship, the degree of autonomy the individual has in interpreting the beliefs and practices of the group, how the group's members are to interact with the Gentile larger surrounding society, and the group's relationship to the land of Israel—all are significant in the expression of Jewish ethnic and religious life.

Jews highly value family and community life, and the Jewish family and community can be a rich source of support. The traditional celebration of the Sabbath, for example, in its fullest expression, sets a whole day apart for family life, worship, and rest. The father presides at the Sabbath meal, and the mother prays over the Sabbath candles to welcome in this very special day. The parents bless the children and have a festive meal that includes many traditional foods and prayers.

Jews celebrate the bris, or circumcision of male children, on the baby's eighth day with great joy, as they do the bar mitzvah, the religious observance of the thirteenth birthday, in which the boy takes on adult responsibility before God and the community. A Jewish worship service must have a minimum of 10 men, a *minyan*, and after the bar mitzvah the boy can be counted as a man for this important purpose. Bat mitzvah celebrations for girls are now increasingly common in the more liberal branches of Judaism.

Judaism recognizes the reality of death in its special treatment of grief and the mourning period. Much in the Jewish faith encourages healthy mourning—from the requirements concerning the preparation of the deceased's body and burial to the 7-day period of intense mourning, a process known as "sitting shivah," in which the grieving family is surrounded by relatives and close friends (Lamm 1969). An interesting aspect of grief and mourning in Judaism is that rabbis state that it is a sin *not* to grieve, but that it is equally a sin to grieve too much or too long. On the anniversary of the death, removing a veil placed over the gravestone ends the grieving period, and loved ones are expected to go on with life as a way of honoring the departed person.

Clinical Implications

General issues that can impinge on diagnosis and treatment of the Jewish patient include the sensitivity toward stereotyping and discrimination and the question of Jewish identity.

The history of discrimination against the Jews dates back to biblical times. For example, Moses was hidden in a basket on the Nile because of a decree to kill Jewish baby boys. As Queen of Persia, Esther hid her Jewish identity, as described in the biblical book of Esther, until the Jewish people were threatened with annihilation, and she risked her life in a successful attempt to save them. The Inquisition in Spain, the pogroms in Russia and Europe, and finally Nazi Germany's attempt to exterminate the Jews in the last century are more recent examples of this oppression.

In the 1940s, 47% of Americans felt "Jews had too much power" (Matthews 1995). In the 1960s, one third "of the population harbored distinctly negative stereotypes of Jews, while as many as another third was tainted by mild evidences of anti-Semitism" (Matthews 1995). Between the 1960s and the 1990s the proportion of Americans agreeing that "Jews have a lot of irritating faults" dropped from 40% to 19%; the proportion who thought "Jews stick together too much" declined from 52% to 40%; and the proportion who believed "Jews use shady practices in business" diminished from 42% to 23% (Matthews 1995). These numbers still speak of a significant degree of bias, and Jews who enter treatment may have a mixture of realistic concerns interwoven with neurotic ones.

The question of Jewish identity is an important one. Some Jews may have a strong sense of their identity as Jews and wear that identity proudly, or they may be very ambivalent about their "Jewishness." Even while knowing that they are without doubt Jewish, they may not quite be able to articulate exactly what that means.

Until a generation or two ago, most Jews were Orthodox, and many Jews today are less observant than their parents or grandparents. Generational tensions focusing on religious allegiance can cause significant distress, as elders see their offspring depart from a culture they consider important to their Jewish identity. Among Jews who are more highly identified with Jewish culture and religion, intermarriage with non-Jews may be seen as a betrayal of Jewish tradition and identity. The preservation of the Jews as a people is seen as being threatened by intermarriage, and such conflicts can be a significant issue in family dynamics.

Although Jews are not evangelistic toward non-Jews, groups within Judaism actively attempt to persuade nonobservant Jews to become more observant. A Jew who decides to become observant, a *"ba'al teshuvah"* (literally, a "master of repentance"), is honored and given encouragement. At the other extreme, those who leave Judaism are threatened with loss of approval from the community. One group that provokes strong feelings within the Jewish community and illustrates this point is the Messianic Jews, or Jews who profess belief that Jesus Christ is the Messiah.

Messianic Jews, or Hebrew Christians, may number as many as 300,000 worldwide. Although many join the general Christian church community, some form congregations in which Jewish culture and tradition are blended with orthodox Christian faith. There are more than 200 Messianic synagogues in the United States and approximately 50 in Israel (Baruch HaShem Synagogue 2003). In celebrating Jewish festivals, members emphasize the symbolic foretelling of the coming of the Messiah. The lamb of the Passover seder dinner represents Jesus, the Lamb of God, and the blood on the door-posts of the Jewish people's homes prior to their exodus from Egypt represents the shed blood of Jesus on the cross that protects believers from the Angel of Death or Judgment. In living their lives as Jews and yet embracing the Christian faith, they assert that they are following biblical Judaism and worshipping the Messiah of the Jews and the Gentiles. They thus challenge the boundaries and the limits of tolerance of the Jewish community regarding Jewish identity.

Some of the literature on psychotherapy with Jews has tried to take into account the effect that the Jews' social history over many generations has had on their values (Cooper 1996; Miller and Lovinger 2000; Rabinowitz 2000). Rotenberg (1987) described the application of Jewish concepts to mental health issues. Strean (1994) wrote an account of psychoanalytic psychotherapy with modern Orthodox Jews in the United States. He suggested that psychoanalytic psychotherapy and Orthodox Judaism are not mutually exclusive and can be mutually enriching. Pliskin (1983) provided a collection of religious statements as an account of the Ultra-Orthodox approach to depression, as reflected in his own work with depressed people in the community. The approach is essentially a cognitive-behavioral one that uses tasks and exercises and presents statements from a range of religious leaders as an antidote to the patient's negative cognitions. The most thorough consideration of the issues in psychodynamic psychotherapy for the religious Jewish patient is to be found in the writings of Spero, from his earlier analyses of religious issues arising in the diagnosis and treatment of religious patients (Spero 1980, 1986) to his more recent evaluation of the attitude toward God in psychotherapy (Spero 1992).

The rest of this chapter will focus primarily on the challenges of attempting to provide psychological services to members of the Ultra-Orthodox community, whose beliefs and practices will be shown to create significant barriers that must be overcome before the community member can embark on psychotherapy. These challenges illustrate clearly the implications of a shared worldview for psychotherapy. Although this population is small and its members are not likely to be seen by most therapists, the following discussion places the issue of a patient's faith and worldview in bold relief as a variable of marked clinical significance.

One of the first hurdles for members of this group is an intrinsic one. How can a religious person seek outside help for distress, when God is the healer of the broken-hearted (Psalms 147:3)—and if not God, then his representative on earth, the rabbi? Further, the actual experiencing of psychological distress or depression may be understood as a sign of a weakness of faith. A second hurdle is the socioreligious one of attachment to the community. A religious Jew is duty bound to listen to his parent, teacher, and rabbi.

Have the parent and the rabbi been consulted, and have they acquiesced to the referral? A third difficulty relates to the type of therapy offered. While psychiatric medications may be perceived as similar to the treatment of physical ailments, the talking cures are more suspect, as they may challenge religious values. The attitudes of Freud (1907/1962) and other psychoanalysts (for example, Reik 1927) toward religion are well known. A more recent contribution to this view from the perspective of rational emotive cognitive therapy was put forth by Ellis (1980), who wrote on the irrationality of being religious. Further, the emphasis of clinicians on psychosexual development and on the centrality of the self rather than the community is seen as a direct challenge to a religious person's spiritual and societal values. The following view of mental health clinicians held by the Ultra-Orthodox community is not unusual: "...the idol worship of psychologists... They are the counsel of sinners, derived from impure sources, and false opinions, foreign to the spirit of Israel" (Shlesinger 1994, quoted by Greenberg and Witztum 2001).

A fourth issue is more external and involves stigma. Marriages within the Ultra-Orthodox community are arranged. Although the final decision to marry is made by the couple, they will only meet a limited number of times. Before they meet, the parents will have made inquiries about the prospective bride or groom and the family. Any illnesses with a genetic component will affect the prospects of all family members, as will the presence of any mental illness or disorder. As a result, families will attempt to deny the existence of a disorder, avoid seeking help unless the need is extreme, and avoid seeking help in public venues that are known to be mental health centers. Those who treat Ultra-Orthodox patients recommend not scheduling members of the community for appointments one after the other to avoid embarrassing meetings that could lead to the termination of the therapy (Margolese 1998).

A fifth issue involves general requests of a religious nature. An Ultra-Orthodox person may be unwilling to sit alone in a room with a person of the opposite sex and so may ask that the door be left open. The Ultra-Orthodox patient will certainly be upset if the therapist is immodestly dressed and may not look at the interviewer during the interview. The patient may ask to be seen by a person of his or her own sex (Rabinowitz 2000) or by a religious, God-fearing therapist. Such requests are not a matter of caprice or individual psychopathology and may reflect the guidance of a religious authority. As stated earlier, the advice of a person's rabbi is definitive on many areas of life. For example, the following statement on the subject of psychiatric treatment was written by Rabbi Moshe Feinstein (1895–1986), the foremost rabbinic authority of his generation:

It is forbidden for a psychiatric patient to go to a psychologist or psychiatrist who is a heretic or atheist. These specialists enquire about the thoughts of a person, and tell him how he should behave, so that one should suspect that occasionally this advice will be against the laws of the Torah, even against the principles of religion, and against matters of modesty. All the healing of psychologists and psychiatrists lies in their words therefore one should take care as they may speak words of heresy and profanity. If they are specialists, and promise the parents that they will not speak against the faith and the law of Torah, one may perhaps rely on them, as they are specialists and should not lie. Therefore, one must seek out a psychologist or psychiatrist who keeps the Torah, but, if this is not possible, one can even go to a heretic or atheist, but it must be stipulated and he must promise not to discuss matters of belief and the Torah with the patient. (Igrot Moshe Yore Deah 2:57)

An external representation of this issue is that Ultra-Orthodox Jews who are referred for treatment often arrive with another person who expects to be present in the interview room and participate in the assessment process. The accompanying person may be a sibling or parent, a teacher or rabbi. Although we initially found that this expectation made us uncomfortable, we have come to understand and accept the presence of others during the interview. As a figure of authority, the accompanying person is accepting responsibility for ensuring that the patient is being put into hands that are capable professionally and respectful religiously. The accompanying person is the spiritual guardian with responsibility for protecting the patient from exposure to nonreligious values (Greenberg 1991; Heilman and Witztum 1994).

An issue of concern of an opposite variety is that referrals from rabbis to therapists whom they trust will do no "religious harm" may cause these therapists to fear a loss of reputation if the patient opts to drop his religious practice. This consideration has the potential to influence the content of their professional work.

Patients' conflicts concerning sexual matters present particular challenges to therapists who treat Ultra-Orthodox patients. Consider the example of a young man who presents with a complaint he calls "defect in the covenant," a euphemism for masturbation. Should the therapist tell him that this behavior is common or even normal? Should he refer him to a rabbi who is understanding and accepting of the behavior? Alternatively, an Ultra-Orthodox man may reveal that he is attracted sexually to men, although he knows that homosexual relations are considered an abomination according to Jewish law (Spero 1986). He also knows that being openly homosexual will lead to him being excluded from his home and community. What is the therapist's role in these cases? Should the therapist help the patient feel comfortable with his sexuality and therefore less connected to his religious roots, help him get in touch with his heterosexual feelings and therefore retain his societal position, or help him understand the importance of both aspects of himself so that any future decision is clearer for him?

The treatment of certain disorders in Ultra-Orthodox patients is especially likely to bring religious content to the fore. Consider as examples obsessive-compulsive disorder (OCD) and social phobia.

Religion is a common theme in OCD in patients who have religion as a central concern in their lives (Greenberg and Shefler 2002). Indeed, Catholics have a special term, *scrupulosity*, for those with excessive religious concerns. Among Ultra-Orthodox Jewish men, the most common concerns are being clean before prayer, leading to compulsive perianal wiping and washing, and concentrated devotion in prayer, leading to repeating prayers over and over. Among women, the most common concern involves the ritual immersion performed a week after menstruation. Their main compulsive behaviors are excessive checking to ensure no staining has occurred during the week after menstruation, checking to see that their bodies are without blemish immediately before immersion, and repeated immersion in the ritual bath until they are convinced they have performed the immersion adequately. Ultra-Orthodox women with OCD may also become preoccupied with the avoidance, cleaning, or hoarding of foods related to the laws of kashruth (Greenberg and Witztum 1994).

The presentation of "religious OCD" involves behaviors that are completely within the context of Ultra-Orthodox Judaism, and the first hurdle for such patients is to recognize that they are not just punctilious or even virtuous but that they have a problem. Baer (2001) quoted William Minichiello, a priest and therapist, who considered his Catholic patients with OCD to have "a totally untheological view of God" (p. 107) and suggested that until they have discussed their concerns thoroughly with their spiritual advisor, they should not embark on exposure therapy. According to Baer (2001), Joseph Ciarrocchi, author of *The Doubting Disease*, noted that such patients often refuse to embark on therapy and suggested a series of maneuvers in cooperation with the patient's priest that would enable the patient to start treatment. For the Ultra-Orthodox patient, however, Jewish law is natural and not excessive. The criteria for disturbance, when religiousness becomes pathological religiosity, are distress or interference with daily functioning, as consistent with the DSM-IV-TR definition of OCD (American Psychiatric Association 2000). The behaviors of OCD are taken from daily religious ritual life in all cases we have seen within the Ultra-Orthodox community, and the impression that these behaviors are exotic is usually a consequence of the therapist's being uninformed. Nevertheless, it is noteworthy that the aspects of religious practice that are selected as the focus for OCD symptoms are often not central to religious life (preprayer cleaning, checking that phylacteries are black) but typical of the symptoms of OCD (Greenberg and Witztum 1994).

Ultra-Orthodox patients with OCD prefer medication to cognitive-behavioral therapy (Greenberg and Shefler 2002). However, a problem arising from the long-term use of medication in an unmarried patient is the duty to tell a potential spouse about the medication and the problem and therefore reveal a source of stigma. On the other hand, cognitive-behavioral therapy requires significant motivation for cooperation throughout and after treatment.

A religious patient who embarks on cognitive-behavioral treatment may question whether a therapist has the authority to advise him, for example, not to repeat prayers, even though the patient is unsure whether he has said them with devotion. If the patient is left feeling he has not prayed at all, it may help for the therapist to meet with the patient's rabbi or at least write to the rabbi to ask if the patient can be permitted not to carry out his repetitive behaviors. Even rabbis associated with the sections of the community known for their punctilious observance of Jewish law are aware of such problems and are typically very encouraging of behavioral approaches. Indeed, exposure methods have a basis in the writings of the Midrash (fifth century) and of Maimonides (twelfth century) (see Greenberg 2001). The following case illustrates how a problem involving repetition of daily prayers was approached by an Ultra-Orthodox rabbi.

> A young man approached his rabbi with a concern about repeating the most important section of the daily prayers, the Shema. The Code of Jewish Law demands that this section be said with "devotion, awe, fear, shaking and trembling" (Code of Jewish Law, Orakh Hayyim, 61:1). Suspecting he had not said this part of the prayer with appropriate attention, had not pronounced the words correctly, or had stray thoughts in his mind at the time, he repeated the first sentence again and again. He also "got stuck" later in the first paragraph and at the end of the third paragraph, another section given special importance. The rabbi told him that he was to stop saying all three paragraphs of the Shema completely for 2 weeks, and then permitted him to replace them in a stepwise fashion, with no repetitions, on a weekly basis. For 6 weeks, he was able to tolerate not saying the most important line of his daily prayers and initially resumed doing so without repetitions. However, he relapsed within the year, and his rabbi then referred him to a psychiatrist for what proved to be a series of medication trials.

This highly respected spiritual leader, known for his guidance on matters of mental health in the Ultra-Orthodox community, had used an approach very similar to that of exposure in behavior therapy. The act of temporary suspension of regular prayer is not within the spectrum of possibilities that can be recommended by a therapist. To understand one of the differences between the rabbi and the therapist in this situation, it is noteworthy that the figure of religious authority is asked a *she'ela* (a question) by those who turn to him, and he replies with a *teshuva* (a definitive answer). His role is not that of an advisor, but of one who gives authoritative direction. The following response from an Ultra-Orthodox rabbi to a question on the subject of religious OCD is insightful:

> Question: A young man is unable to concentrate when he reads the Shema, and repeats each word many times, so as to pronounce each word properly and with exactness, and also out of concern that he did not have the correct concentration on the meaning of the words. And he is in doubt if he had the correct intention of fulfilling the commandment of saying the Shema properly, all of which causes the saying of the Shema to cause him great tension and takes a lot of time.

> Responsum: It is my custom in these cases to tell him that he need only say the words in the prayer book. Even if it seems to him that he has not concentrated, he should continue further (for deep inside he knows what he has said if he understands Hebrew, and even if he does not understand Hebrew, nevertheless his reading is an act of accepting the yoke of the kingdom of heaven). In this way he has fulfilled his duty of saying the Shema. It is forbidden to give him reasons or explanations, for every reason that he is given, he will undermine to contradict and reject completely whatever he was told. When he appears undecided he should be told decisively without any reasons at all. And after all these tricks, one needs a lot of help from Heaven, and may God have mercy on him and send him a complete recovery. (Kanievski 5751, p. 45)

From the emphasis on not entering into discussions on the reasons for the laws, it is clear that Rabbi Kanievski (1899–1985) had seen many such young men. Despite his authority in the Ultra-Orthodox community and the clear instructions he provided, he noted what the young men with this problem tend to do with the advice that is given: they return again and again with their concerns and ultimately find justifications to reject the rabbi's guidance. He had discovered that compulsive reassurance seeking is not helped by reassurance, as noted in all behavioral work. On the subject of excessive time spent cleaning in the toilet before prayers, Rabbi Kanievski wrote:

> On several occasions young men have come to me suffering terribly with this problem... And I know of some young men (now no longer young but in their middle age) whom I really saved from disintegration with this [approach] while one was very stubborn, and always thought he was in the right remained in a state in which he does not pray at all, God forbid, and he is in a very sick state. (Kanievski 5751, p. 53)

There are no data on the effectiveness over time of exposure therapy that has been prescribed by a figure of religious authority. As an alternative approach, if the rabbi gives his approval for the therapy to proceed (rather than ordering its content), the patient is not exonerated from all responsibility and risk. This approach supports treatment intended to overcome anxiety, rather than to offer reassurance, which in our experience is likely to be only transiently beneficial.

Another intriguing example of the interaction between psychopathology and religious law is the problem of social phobia. Anxiety about speaking in public is common in many cultures (Stein et al. 1996), but different societies give different levels of importance to social behaviors. The Code of Jewish Law discourages both social interaction with the opposite sex and "trivial conversation" that diverts time from study of the Torah (see Mishna, Avot 1:5). As a result, a person who immerses himself in religious study and avoids social contact (whether for reasons of extreme anxiety or religious observance) may be perceived as a *zaddik* (a righteous person). However, the reality of Ultra-Orthodox daily life is that social interactions are inevitable. Families are large, and incomes are small, so bedrooms are often shared. School classes are large, and dormitory living is the rule from the teenage years until marriage; even private study is carried out in pairs. It may be that the religious demand for social reticence explains why, despite the actual social pressures of daily life, Ultra-Orthodox patients with an interactional form of social phobia who are pathologically withdrawn and afraid of social contact do not present their social difficulty as their prime problem or even as a feature that requires change (Greenberg and Brom 2001).

In contrast, individuals with social phobia of the performance variety in the Ultra-Orthodox community may seek treatment for two types of difficulties. One is speaking publicly before an audience, a situation reserved for the *talmid haham* (literally, "a wise pupil"). A talmid haham is one who is respected for his wisdom in religious matters and his correct moral behavior. As a mark of his standing, he will be called on at special gatherings, including weddings and circumcisions, to say words of the Torah. If the man is prevented from accepting as a result of extreme anxiety, he will be losing an opportunity to bring his ideas to a wider audience than those who read his writings and will not participate in the ultimate public accolade for a respected spiritual leader.

The second setting concerns leading religious ceremonies, such as the thrice-daily prayers or saying the blessing over the public reading of the Torah. Although patients with these problems do not have difficulties saying blessings in front of the family (such as the *kiddush* and *havdala* ceremonies said over wine at the beginning and end of the Sabbath), they do experience anxiety and avoidance if guests are present.

Mr. B. is 48 years old and is married with eight children. He has spent all his life in Jewish studies and has worked on editing ancient manuscripts. "I have a phobia that cripples me, although I function. It affects me when I appear in public. If not for this problem, I would have opened a school. When I am writing, I have no fear." Mr. B. is a successful and admired person in his community, but he feels he is unable to do what he really wants.

Ever since he can remember, Mr. B. has had a fear of appearing in public. At wedding meals, he leaves before the grace after meals to avoid being asked to recite a blessing. In synagogue he avoids being asked to read the *haftara* (public reading of a chapter of the Bible), and he can only lead the prayers in a synagogue where he is unknown. Despite being a very meticulous Ultra-Orthodox Jew, he avoids going to the synagogue on Saturday afternoon, as the crowd is small and the chance of being called to read the Torah is high. He becomes anxious before saying the blessing for wine on Friday night with his family and very anxious if strangers are present. When his daughters become pregnant he starts to become anxious, because if a son is born, there will be a public circumcision, and he will be expected to take a role in the ceremony. His parents, "May they live many years," are alive, and he finds himself thinking about the eventuality of their deaths, when he will have to lead public prayers for a whole year and say Kaddish.

His fear in all of these situations is that he will blush. Blushing starts a chain reaction in him. His voice chokes, and his legs tremble. He then feels sure that people are aware of his difficulty and stare at him, and he blushes more. As a result of his difficulties, he feels frustrated that his intellectual ability has never been transmitted verbally and that it is only accessible to those who read his books. In the past he sought a range of help. He first went to rabbis for advice, then to Kabbalists for blessings and remedies ("sorcerers" he added with a wry smile). He explains that his Lithuanian background did not really encourage him to seek help from Kabbalists, but after the advice of his rabbi had not helped, it was worth a try.

To someone outside the community, the scope of this patient's problem may seem very restricted. The implications of the problem, however, are much broader, as both public prayers and meals with strangers are integral features of communal religious life. To avoid either creates religious conflict. Treatment for a phobia of speaking publicly is recognized within the community, and group treatment with an emphasis on relaxation even exists. Successful treatment of the phobia of leading prayers is more complex, as, like religious OCD, it involves the correct pronunciation of the actual prayers, and the patient may consider the therapist unauthorized to encourage him to continue the public prayer or blessing despite stumbling over the words. As a rule, however, the religious motivation is usually not in evidence, and the concern is social—a fear of being shamed. Nevertheless, we have found that, if the patient has not already discussed the religious aspects with his rabbi, he should do so to ascertain whether he can proceed despite feeling he may have slurred or stumbled over the words. Using exposure in vivo, we have constructed a hierarchy of difficult situations that the patient undertakes. If the patient is to be asked to recite some prayers before the therapist and invited strangers, it can help to ask the rabbi if such practice recitals are permissible.

It is worth noting that while the restrictions imposed by a social phobia of the performance type allow the Ultra-Orthodox community to support its treatment, treating a more generalized interactional social phobia may be religiously unacceptable. In addition, our experience is that referrals of men with social phobia from the Ultra-Orthodox community are uncommon, and referrals of women are nonexistent. We suggest that women are not referred because the religious attitude toward modesty in women prevents a social phobia from being experienced as a problem. This explanation is consistent with the finding of El-Islam (1994) of very few cases of agoraphobia and social phobia in a sample of Muslim women in a psychiatric outpatient clinic in Qatar. He commented: "Being bound to the home, which is a sign of severe agoraphobia in the West, is a sign of virtue in a Muslim housewife; the Koran (holy book of Muslims) addresses women in the verse 'stay in your homes and do not misbehave like the early pagans!'" (El-Islam 1994, p. 139).

Variations of Therapeutic Encounters

This chapter has addressed several unique aspects of clinical work involving Ultra-Orthodox Jewish patients and a Jewish psychiatrist quite knowledgeable about Jewish faith and practice.

In some instances, Jewish psychiatrists of one subdivision of Judaism may have as much difficulty understanding a Jewish patient of another subdivision as they might have of understanding a non-Jewish patient. There are other variations in clinical work in which the Jewish worldview is important.

Non-Jewish clinicians who are treating a Jewish patient should recognize a sensitivity toward prejudice that some patients may demonstrate. This perspective should be explored with attention to the clinical data on which this perspective is based. The non-Jewish clinician may need to pay extra attention to developing a trusting patient-clinician relationship in such encounters. Non-Jewish psychiatrists will need to identify and manage any tendency within themselves toward the stereotyping of Jewish patients. As with all ethnic, cultural, and faith traditions, it is vital to separate the psychopathology of the Jewish patient from healthy ethnicity. There may be occasions in which a non-Jewish psychiatrist is preferred by the Jewish patient, who may believe that someone outside the faith and tradition may be more objective in the treatment relationship.

A Jewish psychiatrist who treats non-Jewish patients will have a parallel task of considering the effect of his or her worldview in the assessment of the patient. If the Jewish psychiatrist is not practicing the Jewish faith, he or she may have to be careful to thoroughly evaluate the religious ideation of a devout patient. On the other hand, a psychiatrist who is a nonpracticing Jew may be particularly attuned to the worldview of the secular patient who has no particular faith tradition.

Collaboration With Faith Communities

Therapists who work with Ultra-Orthodox patients must understand the difference between the written codes of law and the personal, authoritative statements made by rabbis. As an example, in Ultra-Orthodox society no written texts permit masturbation. If a young man consults his rabbi on this subject, he is likely to be advised to study more and marry soon. If he returns to his rabbi and is still in great distress, he will be guided to focus on other things and not allow himself to get overly upset. While he will be encouraged to try to abstain, he may also be discouraged from ascribing too much importance to the behavior. The rabbi will intuitively emphasize the diminution of guilt, although he will never say, "That's fine, you go ahead and do it whenever you want." The rabbi will also recognize when the sense of guilt is persisting and damaging to daily life beyond what the young man normally experiences. At this point, the rabbi may encourage the patient to go to a therapist to discuss or receive medication to address the patient's crippling distress. If such a patient seeks help before consulting his rabbi, the therapist and patient may decide he should first get his rabbi's agreement. If, as a first response, the rabbi prefers to send the patient to a counselor within the community, the professional therapist should accept this decision rather than challenge the authority of the rabbi (Buchbinder 1994).

It is important to understand that whatever passed between the rabbi and the patient was unique to that interaction. If the patient told the therapist about the rabbi's statements, the therapist cannot conclude that the rabbi's pronouncement constitutes rewriting of the law codes nor should the therapist present these statements as guidance to other patients. The therapist can only encourage each individual patient to seek rabbinical guidance himself. The therapist must accept his or her lack of control over the situation. If the patient returns from a visit to a rabbi having been urged to study harder, the therapist will no doubt feel frustrated. It may be tempting to suggest that the patient visit a more flexible (Reform vs. Orthodox) rabbi, as did Baer (2001) in treating religious patients with OCD. However, this course of action entails the risk of trying to place one's own authority over that of the rabbi. Uninvited, and because of motives that are his or her own, the therapist is then interfering with the value system of the patient. In most cases, the patient will drop out of psychotherapy owing to the growing clash between the authority of his religious mentor and his psychotherapist.

References

American Jewish Committee: 2002 Annual Survey of American Jewish Opinion. New York, American Jewish Committee, 2003. Available at http://www.ajc.org/InTheMedia/PubSurveys.asp?did=734. Accessed March 4, 2003.

American Psychiatric Association: Diagnostic and Statistical Manual of Mental Disorders, 4th Edition, Text Revision. Washington, DC, American Psychiatric Association, 2000

Ash R: The Top 10 of Everything. New York, DK Publishing, 1997, pp 160–161

Baer L: The Imp of the Mind: Exploring the Silent Epidemic of Obsessive Bad Thoughts. New York, Dutton, 2001

Baruch HaShem Synagogue: What is Messianic Judaism? Dallas, TX, Baruch HaShem Synagogue, 2003. Available at: http://www.baruchhashem.com/menus/menusmj.html. Accessed March 6, 2003.

Buchbinder JT: The professional credo of an ultra-orthodox psychotherapist. Isr J Psychiatry Relat Sci 31:183–188, 1994

Cooper H: "The cracked crucible": Judaism and mental health, in Psychiatry and Religion: Context, Consensus and Controversies. Edited by Bhugra D. London, Routledge, 1966, pp 65–81

El-Islam MF: Cultural aspects of morbid fears in Qatari women. Soc Psychiatry Psychiatr Epidemiol 29:137–140, 1994

Ellis A: Psychotherapy and atheistic values—a response to AE Bergin's "Psychotherapy and religious values." J Consult Clin Psychology 48:635–639, 1980

Freud S: Obsessive acts and religious practices (1907), in The Standard Edition of the Complete Psychological Works of Sigmund Freud, Vol 9. Translated and edited by Strachey J. London, Hogarth Press, 1962, pp 115–127

Greenberg D: Is psychotherapy possible with unbelievers? The care of the ultraorthodox community. Isr J Psychiatry Relat Sci 28:19–30, 1991

Greenberg D: A religious psychiatrist's ethnographic self-report. Am J Psychother 55:564–576, 2001

Greenberg D, Brom D: Nocturnal hallucinations in ultra-orthodox Jewish Israeli men. Psychiatry 64:81–90, 2001

Greenberg D, Shefler G: Obsessive compulsive disorder in ultra-orthodox Jewish patients: a comparison of religious and non-religious symptoms. Psychol Psychother 75:123–130, 2002

Greenberg D, Witztum E: The influence of cultural factors on obsessive compulsive disorder: religious symptoms in a religious society. Isr J Psychiatry Relat Sci 31:211–220, 1994

Greenberg, D, Witztum E: Sanity and Sanctity: Mental Health Work Among the Ultra-Orthodox in Jerusalem. New Haven, CT, Yale University Press, 2001

Heilman SC, Witztum E: Patients, chaperons and healers: enlarging the therapeutic encounter. Soc Sci Med 39:133–143, 1994

Information Please Almanac: Top Ten Organized Religions of the World. Available at: http://www.infoplease.com/ipa/A0904108.html. Accessed May 7, 2004.

Jewish Reconstructionist Federation: What is a Reconstructionist Jew? Elkins Park, PA, Jewish Reconstructionist Federation, 2000. Available at: http://jrf.org/recon/whois.html. Accessed March 4, 2003.

Kanievski Y: Etzot Vehadrachot [Advice and Guidance]. Monsey, NY, Greenwald, 5751 (Hebrew)

Lamm M: The Jewish Way in Death and Mourning. New York, Jonathan David, 1969

Margolese HC: Engaging in psychotherapy with the Orthodox Jew: a critical review. Am J Psychother 52:37–53, 1998

Matthews T: The Changing Nature of Denominational Life. Winston-Salem, NC, Wake Forest University, Religion Department, 1995. Available at: http://www.wfu.edu/~matthetl/perspectives/thirtythree.html. Accessed March 6, 2003.

Miller L, Lovinger RJ: Psychotherapy with Conservative and Reform Jews, in Handbook of Psychotherapy and Religious Diversity. Edited by Richards PS, Bergin AE. Washington, DC, American Psychological Association, 2000, pp 259–286

North American Jewish Data Bank: National Jewish Population Survey 1990. Waltham, MA, North American Jewish Data Bank, 2001. Available at: http://www.jewishdatabank.org/index.cfm?page=50. Accessed June 8, 2004.

Pliskin Z: Gateway to happiness. Jerusalem, Aish HaTorah, 1983

Rabinowitz A: Psychotherapy with Orthodox Jews, in Handbook of Psychotherapy and Religious Diversity. Edited by Richards PS, Bergin AE. Washington, DC, American Psychological Association, 2000, pp 237–258

Reik T: Dogma and Compulsions. New York, Greenwood, 1927

Rotenberg M: Re-biographing and Deviance: Psychotherapeutic Narrativism and the Midrash. New York, Praeger, 1987

Schorsch I: The Core Values of Conservative Judaism. February 8, 1995. Jewish Virtual Library. Available at: http://www.us-israel.org/jsource/Judaism/conservative_values.html. Accessed March 4, 2003.

Spero MH: Judaism and Psychology: Halakhic Perspectives. New York, Ktav/Yeshiva University, 1980

Spero MH: Handbook of Psychotherapy and Jewish Ethics: Halakhic Perspectives on Professional Values and Techniques. New York, Feldheim, 1986

Spero MH: Religious Objects as Psychological Structures: A Critical Integration of Object Relations Theory, Psychotherapy, and Judaism. Chicago, IL, University of Chicago, 1992

Stein MB, Walker JR, Forde DR: Public-speaking fears in a community sample: prevalence, impact on functioning, and diagnostic classification. Arch Gen Psychiatry 53:169–174, 1996

Strean H: Psychotherapy with the Orthodox Jew. Northvale, NJ, Jason Aronson, 1994

Ultra-Orthodox Judaism. From Wikipedia, the Free Encyclopedia, 2003. Available at: http://en.wikipedia.org/wiki/Ultra-Orthodox_Judaism. Accessed March 4, 2003.

Union of American Hebrew Congregations: What is Reform Judaism? New York, Union of American Hebrew Congregations, 2002. Available at: http://rj.org/ whatisrj.shtml. Accessed March 4, 2003.

CHAPTER 8

Muslims

Yousef Abou-Allaban, M.D.

Introduction

Islam, which literally means "submission," began in 610 A.D. with an encounter between the prophet Muhammad and an angel on a mountain just outside the city of Mecca in the Arabian Peninsula when Muhammad was 40 years old. For the next 23 years of his life, Muslims believe, Muhammad gradually received the Holy Koran through the Angel Gabriel, who delivered the words from God Himself (Husain 1998). The first command that he received focused on acquiring knowledge and encouraging people to read. It states, "Read in the name of your Lord Who created. He created man from a clot. Read and your Lord is Most Honorable, Who taught (to write) with the pen." (Koran, Chapter 96, Verses 1–4) (Pickthall 1984, p. 723). The Koran explains that Islam is the religion of all prophets before Muhammad in that they all submitted their will to one God. Muhammad was the last in a long line of prophets stretching back through Jesus, Moses, and Abraham to Adam. Islam shares with the major religions of Christianity and Judaism a focus on these links between human beings and their Creator.

As Muhammad began to proclaim the revelation that there is only one God deserving of reverence and obedience, he and his followers were persecuted and tortured by the clans of Mecca. Because of this persecution, Muhammad and his followers migrated in 623 A.D. to the nearby city of Medina. In this oasis town the Prophet and his followers built the first Islamic society, and, after a series of hard-fought battles with the Meccans, they finally returned to Mecca, the site of the early revelations (Al-Mubarakpuri 1995).

If the Koran is the constitution of Islam, then Muhammad's life represents the practical application of the Koran. Through his everyday kindness, patience, and wisdom, Muhammad demonstrated to other believers how they should live their lives as Muslims. A former trader, he was known for his honesty and fairness; before receiving his call to prophethood, he earned the nickname Al-Amin, or the Trustworthy, and was called on to arbitrate among rival clans in Mecca. Later, when he reigned as a spiritual and political leader in Medina, the prophet maintained a humble existence, dwelling in simple mud-walled apartments and assisting all petitioners who came to him.

The Prophet died in 633 A.D., 23 years after the Angel Gabriel commanded him to "Read!" A successor was chosen to head the young Islamic state, and the religion quickly spread to three continents. The Islamic empire that followed reached a level of prosperity that stimulated and sustained invention, as citizens enjoyed a degree of safety and security that had been absent for many centuries.

Core Beliefs and Practices

Islamic law, or *shari'a*, which guides the believer in every aspect of his or her life ranging from marriage to prayer to trade, is derived primarily from two sources: the Koran and the prophetic traditions known as *hadith* (plural: *ahadith*). Muslims consider the Koran to be the verbatim word of Allah. In Muhammad's lifetime, the Koran was written down and memorized. It is viewed as a text by which Allah speaks directly to the believer and offers guidance for life and the hereafter. It is not written in a narrative fashion, as in the Christian Gospels or the Jewish Pentateuch. The prophetic traditions, or *ahadith,* are the record of some of Muhammad's activities during his lifetime. From the recollections of family and friends, Muslims today know such things as how the Prophet washed himself and how he personally interacted with his grandchildren. In addition to these private matters, the *ahadith* relay how he conducted his political life, solved disputes among his followers, and offered spiritual advice.

A Muslim is anyone who believes in and practices the "five pillars" of Islam. The first pillar is the declaration of faith that Allah (God) is the only one worthy of worship and that Muhammad is his messenger. Second, Muslims perform five daily prayers either individually or in a congregation. Third, during the month of Ramadan, Muslims refrain from food, drink, or sexual intercourse during the daylight. Fourth, Muslims have a mandatory alms tax of 2.5% of the believer's savings and investments, paid annually to the poor, as well as to support religious and educational purposes. Fifth and finally, a pilgrimage to Mecca is required once in the lifetime for every Muslim who can afford the trip financially and physically. Each year pilgrims find themselves in a literal sea of humanity, surrounded on all sides by nearly 2 million Muslims hailing from nearly every nation on the planet.

About 1.5 billion people currently identify themselves as Muslims. With Muslims now present in nearly every country around the globe, ranging from South Africa to Singapore to Brazil, Islam encompasses or influences an enormous number of highly varied cultures. Despite this fact, the misconception that most Muslims are Arabs remains widespread in the United States. In reality, Arabs represent only about 14% of Muslims worldwide and about 25% of the American Muslim community (Alam 2002). Indonesia is home to more Muslims than all 22 Arab countries combined. One of Islam's great strengths is its ability to absorb and maintain local culture. A Muslim may engage in all aspects of his or her native culture except those that are clearly delineated by Islam as prohibited (for example, the prohibition on alcohol).

An estimated 8 million Muslims live in the United States (Council on American-Islamic Relations 2001). The scene at the Islamic Society of Boston Mosque in Cambridge, Massachusetts, sheds some light on the diversity of Muslims living in the United States today. Every Friday afternoon nearly 1,000 Muslims, representing more than 40 different nationalities, attend the congregational Friday prayers. The majority of Muslims currently living in the United States may be grouped into one of two categories: 1) Muslim immigrants and their descendents and 2) nonimmigrant Americans of varying races who have converted to, or "embraced," Islam. American-born Muslims include African American Muslims, American Muslims born to immigrant parents, and converts to Islam.

African Americans compose the largest Muslim ethnic group in North America. They began arriving in large numbers through the African slave trade in the seventeenth century. Most of those early comers gave up their religion, just as they were forced to give up their other freedoms (Hedayat-diba 2000). It was not until the twentieth century that African American interest in Islam was revived. In 1930 Elijah Muhammad established the Nation of Islam and advocated a separate black nation where African Americans could govern themselves. In the early teaching of the Nation of Islam, white people were described as devils, and God and Prophet Muhammad were described as black. These claims, along with other extreme aspects of the Nation's ideology, prompted Islamic scholars to question whether the Nation of Islam truly preached Islam. After the death of Elijah Muhammad in 1975, the Nation of Islam underwent a major division. Elijah's son, Warith Deen Muhammad, led a majority of the followers away from the heterodox teachings of the Nation of Islam and into the mainstream practice of Sunni Islam. A minority of Nation of Islam followers remained under the leadership of Louis Farrakhan.

American Muslims born to immigrant parents suffer from tremendous cultural stress and the resulting conflict (Rashed 2000). Immigrant parents usually impose values and forms of discipline from their country of origin that in many circumstances conflict with American values and forms of discipline. Conflict is sharper when one parent follows a different religion.

American converts to Islam are small in number. They often have difficulty distinguishing between the cultural aspects of the immigrant Muslims' practices and pure Islamic teaching. This difficulty can confuse them as they begin to practice their new faith.

Muslim immigrants came to the United States in three different waves. The first wave, in the late nineteenth century, mostly constituted individuals and families from the Middle East and South Asia who sought a better economic life in the United States. The middle of the twentieth century witnessed a second wave, which again included South Asians and Arabs from the Middle East and consisted of professionals and university students who remained in the United States after their education (Erickson and al-Timimi 2001) and some persons who were fleeing repressive political systems in their home countries. The third wave, which began in the 1970s and currently continues, is largely composed of Muslim students, professionals, and entrepreneurs from many different countries who are seeking opportunities in the United States. A new wave seems to have emerged in the last 10 years. Although this most recent wave of Muslim immigrants is not well defined, the majority seems to consist of refugees from Afghanistan, Bosnia, Kosovo, Somalia, and other war-torn countries. Many of these immigrants are experiencing the effects of trauma. As evidence of this trend, the International Institute of Boston, which has been resettling refugees and assisting new arrivals for the past 80 years, reported a major shift in their target population in recent years, with Muslims currently accounting for 65% of the agency's clients (W. Eqman, director of the International Institute of Boston, personal communication, July 2002).

An enormous disparity exists between the current Muslim understanding of mental illnesses, which is often marked by stigma, and the religious texts and past practices of Muslims (Zareek 1993). The Koran speaks about numerous psychological phenomena, including anger, obsessive thinking, panic, and phobias, and the Prophet Muhammad offered a variety of advice on how to handle these phenomena. Many of Islam's most illustrious physicians and scholars also treated and wrote about emotional conditions. For example, Ibn Sina (known to the West as Avicenna, b. ca. 980 A.D.) wrote an entire treatise on melancholia; Muhammad Al-Ghazali (d. 1111 A.D.) described conditioned reflexes and learning; and Al-Balkhi classified neurosis into four types and depression into three types (Badri 2000).

Given this rich textual and historical background, why should a contemporary Muslim be reluctant to acknowledge mental health as a legitimate and necessary concern? One answer may lie with the fragmentation of Islamic civilization over time. The thirteenth century witnessed a peak of Islamic culture, when scholarship in all fields of knowledge flourished. In the year 1258 A.D., however, the Mongol army destroyed Baghdad, the capital of the Islamic empire, and with it destroyed a host of key educational institutions. In the nineteenth century, when Muslim lands were divided and colonized by different Western countries, Muslim people were exposed to Western conceptions of mental illness. The Freudian school of psychoanalysis carried with it a negative view of religion. Those who established the new field of psychiatry in Muslim countries were Western-trained psychiatrists who not only carried the view that religion was a hindrance, not a help, to mental health but also attempted to apply Western methods in a very different cultural context (Shehu 2002).

Through these periods of sociopolitical upheaval, many Muslims lost hold of the guidance that their religious tradition offered them in coping with mental health difficulties, and the roles of the Muslim and Western countries seemed to have been reversed: In the medieval era, Muslims had benefited from hospitals and mental health treatment, while Europeans had languished in the Dark Ages. In the era of colonialism, however, Europe was developing new treatments for mental illnesses, while Muslims reverted to blaming these illnesses on witches, devils, or curses from God.

Clinical Implications

Islam teaches that when one gets angry, one should immediately change one's physical position. If the angry person is standing, he should sit. If he is sitting, then he should lie down. If the person is still angry, he or she should offer a short supplication for taking refuge in God from the anger. After this supplication, the person should make a ritual ablution and then offer two or more cycles of prayer. The water of the ablution is meant to literally "cool" the anger, while the prayer helps to refocus the mind and restore a feeling of humility. The Prophet strongly counseled against becoming angry and frequently reminded people of the negative consequences of anger (Al-Sanee'a 2000).

The Prophet encouraged daily meditation (similar to a cognitive-behavioral therapy) to minimize day-to-day stress (El-Kadi 1989). Muslims are to set aside 15 to 20 minutes every morning and evening to read or recite the Koran or repeat some of the supplications from the prophetic tradition. When faced with a particular anxiety, they are to pray two extra cycles of prayer and then ask for God's help through the following supplication:

"O God I seek refuge in Thee from worry and grief, and I seek refuge in Thee from helplessness and laziness, and I seek refuge in Thee from miserliness and cowardice, and from the burden of debts, and from being overpowered by others."

Muslims do not believe that human beings carry a burden of original sin. In the Koranic account of the story of Adam and Eve, the couple sins against God but then repents and is forgiven. Every child born into the world is thus considered to be in a state of *fitrah*, or moral purity, in complete submission to God. After committing a sin, a person is encouraged to turn in repentance to God to seek His mercy. The Koran reinforces this point, stating: "Say, O My servants who have been prodigal to their own hurt! Despair not of the mercy of Allah, Who forgives all the sins. Lo! He is the forgiving, the Merciful. Turn unto him repentant, and surrender unto him" (Koran 39:53) (Pickthall 1984, p. 499). This emphasis on repentance and mercy may provide relief to patients who may be experiencing overwhelming feelings of guilt related to obsessive-compulsive disorder, severe depression, or even mild psychosis.

Suicidal thinking is uncommon in the Muslim mind, and the suicide rate is extremely low in Muslim communities worldwide (Hedayat-diba 2000). This relatively low incidence, however, should not discourage the clinician from inquiring about suicide, albeit with a slightly modified strategy. A Muslim patient often gives a negative answer if asked directly if he or she is considering suicide, even though the patient has severe depression and may be in urgent need of hospitalization. It is important to be aware of this pattern, because guilt can prevent the person from engaging in treatment. A possible way around this roadblock is to ask if the depressed patient "wishes he [or she] were dead." The answer to this question may afford a better means of assessing the patient's level of desperation and potential for a suicide attempt. Since more than one session may be needed before a Muslim patient agrees to take medication, it is important to engage the patient in intensive psychotherapy as soon as possible. The following case describes a young student who had suicidal thoughts for an extended period of time:

> Ms. S. was a 19 year-old college student who was a practicing Muslim. She was born and raised in the United States to parents of Pakistani origin and was an honor student in high school. However, she started feeling depressed a few weeks after arriving at college and did very poorly in the first semester, failing three of her four courses. She developed a strong sense of guilt and shame over her failure. One of her close friends insisted that she should see a psychiatrist, but she refused to see anyone who was not a Muslim. By the time she first saw a Muslim psychiatrist 3 months later she was severely depressed and isolated and had lost more than 15 of her original 115 lbs. Early in the interview she denied any suicidal or homicidal ideation, as well as any

personal or family history of psychiatric illness. Toward the end of the first conversation with the psychiatrist, however, she burst into tears and expressed overwhelming guilt over suicidal thoughts about throwing herself into the river. She questioned the strength of her faith and whether she was a good Muslim. She was aware that Islam does not allow suicide, but she felt worthless and considered her depression a punishment from God. After three appointments she eventually agreed to take an antidepressant. She took a year off from college, during which she returned home to live with her family. A year later, she resumed school, feeling much better and still taking an antidepressant.

Although the Koran acknowledges that a human being may reach a level of extreme desperation, God advises against committing suicide: "… and kill not one another (nor yourself). Lo! Allah is ever merciful unto you" (Koran 4:29) (Pickthall 1984, p. 79). It is unfortunate, however, that the issue of suicide among Muslims is frequently reduced to statements like "suicide is not allowed in Islam" and that those who do commit suicide will burn in hellfire for their sin. While Islamic law does indeed prohibit the wrongful taking of life, including one's own, the Koran and other sources in fact offer a far more nuanced look at this issue.

The family of a person who commits suicide may experience tremendous guilt and fear that the person will be punished in hellfire. However, Islam teaches that someone in an advanced state of depression or psychosis who attempts to take his or her own life may not have the clear state of mind required to make such a choice. The prophet distinguished three types of states that interfere with accountability for one's actions: 1) being asleep; 2) being *al-majnoon* (an Arabic term that indicates a disturbed state of reality such as acute psychosis, delirium, or advanced depression); and 3) being incapable of handling financial affairs (a state experienced by very young and very old persons).

Islam offers a desperate person help in overcoming hopeless feelings through a cognitive approach based on the Koranic assertion that God is closer to a human being than his "jugular vein" (Koran 50:16). That is, the scriptures reassure the troubled person that he or she is not alone and helpless but rather has access to the One who has complete control over his or her existence and, therefore, over the state of despair. Just as God can help the insomniac sleep, so is He able to lift the cloud of hopelessness that engulfs the depressed person. Further, Muslims believe that affliction is sent in order to test human beings and increase their level of faith. Each hardship— even, according to prophetic tradition, a pinprick on the foot—may lead to a higher level of faith. This point is particularly salient, since closeness to God is the final goal of the Muslim.

The afflicted individual may also request that friends and family pray for his or her recovery. If the person reaches a stage of utter bleakness, he or she may recite the following prophetic prayer: "O Allah keep me alive as long as living is beneficial to me, and end my life as long as death is better for me." Through the prayer, then, the afflicted person is able to voice his or her desire for death, while still recognizing that ownership of his or her life ultimately lies in God's hands. Islam encourages believers in any of these states to seek professional help.

During the time of the Prophet, the Arabs of Mecca were accustomed to drinking alcohol. Because some of the early Muslims arrived at the mosque for prayer in a state of intoxication, the first teachings about alcohol prohibited praying while drunk. Later, verses that forbade any consumption of alcohol gradually appeared as reminders to believers of the value of the human mind and the importance of being fully conscious. The gradual revelation of the verses pertaining to the prohibition on alcohol or illicit intoxicants in Islam is testimony to the fact that the Koran acknowledges how difficult it can be to reach and maintain sobriety (El-Kadi and El-Kadi 1997).

Substance abuse is less prevalent among Muslims than among non-Muslims. Most Muslim substance abusers encountered by mental health professionals are either converts or nonpracticing Muslims. Self-identified Muslims may deny that they are using or abusing substances, and it may take several sessions before they are willing to admit this activity to the clinician.

In the treatment process, Islam may provide a familiar framework in which to become sober. In many parts of the United States, there is a group called *Mullati Islami* that is similar to Alcoholics Anonymous, but with an Islamic reinterpretation of the 12 steps. The clinician may help the recovering substance abuser by encouraging resumption of Islamic practices, such as the five daily prayers and Friday congregational prayer. Religious counseling by the local imam may strengthen the patient's motivation to stay sober.

A 50-year-old Muslim restaurant owner came for treatment of a 15-year history of alcohol abuse and pathological gambling. Although he had functioned fairly well, he had become troubled by the amount of money he spent every month on gambling and wine. Several previous attempts to stop both activities, including brief trials of psychotherapy, had failed. He had been in the United States for 25 years, was not a practicing Muslim, and was married to an American-born Christian. However, he accepted a referral to a Muslim psychiatrist from his Muslim primary care physician. The psychiatrist diagnosed a moderate level of depression and recommended that an antidepressant be added to the patient's regimen of naltrexone. The psychiatrist also offered to see the patient twice a month, when he would report on the number of lottery tickets he bought each week and the number of drinks he consumed each day. The psychiatrist encouraged him to start going to the mosque for the Friday congregational prayer, on the condition that he would not drink for at least 48 hours beforehand. His visits to the mosque increased in frequency, whereas his drinking decreased dramatically and his gambling ceased altogether after 3 months. When the Muslim holy month of Ramadan started that year, he committed himself to fasting for the entire month and planned a visit to Mecca during Ramadan to conduct *'Umra*, a ritual "smaller pilgrimage" to Mecca outside the official pilgrimage season of hajj. By the end of Ramadan his drinking and gambling had stopped completely. He continued to see the psychiatrist for bimonthly visits for almost a year without any relapse. He stopped taking both naltrexone and the antidepressant and has remained sober without a relapse for more than 2 years.

This case illustrates the potential for helping a patient achieve sobriety by encouraging him to practice his faith.

It can help grieving Muslims to remember that Islam accepts death as part of the journey of life. Muslims believe that after death, the individual will spend time in the grave and enter a transitional state, known as *barzakh* (literally meaning "barrier"), and ultimately be resurrected on the Day of Judgment. On hearing that someone has died, a Muslim traditionally says: "Verily we come from God and to Him we shall return." This statement is a reminder that our lives do not belong to us, but rather to God, and that we will all inevitably face Him one day. Reading or reciting passages from the Koran can have a calming effect by further reminding the individual about God's promise of the next life.

Muslims believe in the presence of another category of created beings called *jinn* (evil jinn are called devils) (see Chapter 72 of the Koran) (Pickthall 1984, pp. 658–659). Muslims believe that devils may distract believers from doing good actions through demonic "whispering" or *waswasa*. However, there is no mention in the Koran of jinn being responsible for the mental illnesses that inflict human beings, a common belief among uneducated Muslims. Recent Muslim immigrants in particular may interpret auditory and visual hallucinations as communication with jinn. They may also interpret odd speech or behavior as evidence that the jinn have possessed someone and are using the person's body as a vessel through which to speak and act. The purported treatment for this condition is to literally "beat the jinn" out of the patient. Clinicians may find it difficult to differentiate between psychotic symptoms (such as a patient's saying "I hear or see the devil who ordered me to do so and so") and the notion that the devil can influence an individual's behavior through whispering.

Variations of Clinical Encounters

Non-Muslim clinicians who treat Muslim patients need a high level of sensitivity as well as background information on how a Muslim might participate in the treatment process. The following strategies are often helpful:

1. *Involve family members in the treatment process whenever possible, if appropriate.* Muslims tend to be family- and community-oriented, even when they live in individualistic societies such as the United States. Patients may prefer to bring another person along to a treatment session; if a family member is not available, a close friend may serve as a substitute.

2. *Assess the level of education and religiosity.* Well-educated practicing Muslims tend to feel that mental illness carries less stigma than do less well-educated Muslims. However, it is worthwhile to spend a few minutes assuring the patient that mental illnesses are neither a curse from God nor the result of the evil eye or the person's lack of faith. The clinician can remind the Muslim patient that the Koran and the prophetic traditions discuss mental illnesses and encourage their treatment.

3. *Emphasize the biological basis of mental illnesses and that medication may be able to relieve symptoms.* In my practice, I often mention diabetes as an analogy to depression or anxiety.

4. *Use exploratory-directive methods rather than the exploratory-reflective methods to solicit information* (Al Abdul-Jabbar and Al-Issa 2000). An exploratory-directive approach utilizes the familiar "parent-child" mode of interaction and allows the therapist to assume parental authority to direct, advise, provide care, and at times criticize. It also allows active manipulation of the cognitive process and the patient's behavior. Exploratory-reflective approaches allow the therapist to encourage the patient's interaction and reflection on the cause of his ailment, but these approaches are appropriate for fewer Muslim patients. These patients may not fully understand the role of the psychologist or social worker. If, for example, a psychiatrist refers a patient to someone else for therapy, the patient may assume that the clinician is not skillful enough to provide them with treatment. Referring clinicians are well advised to discuss the roles of the patient and therapist at the beginning of treatment to avoid potential misunderstandings.

A newly practicing Muslim therapist or psychiatrist may feel intimidated about disclosing his or her own religion. These feelings arise mainly because of concerns that the negative stereotypes that exist about Islam will lead the patient to establish a negative transference early in the treatment. The clinician's Muslim practices may be evident—a practicing Muslim has to pray daily, take time off for the obligatory Friday prayer, fast daily for a whole month once a year, and so on. The newly practicing Muslim clinician may fear that the patient will cease treatment because he or she will object to the therapist's Islamic heritage and may assume that the therapist's religion will influence his or her points of view on certain subjects.

A Muslim therapist may be able to help a Muslim patient develop trust more rapidly. This shared background can be an important advantage in engaging individuals from immigrant populations, who may have a higher level of paranoia than others. However, Muslims make up an extremely diverse group and include Muslims born and raised in the United States, who often engage easily in treatment. It would be just as difficult for me as a Muslim psychiatrist (of Middle Eastern background) to understand a Muslim patient of South Asian origin who has just immigrated to the United States as it would for a non-Muslim psychiatrist to understand this patient.

Personal Observations

My own experience as a private practitioner in interacting with Muslims and non-Muslims has been mixed. Some patients have elected not to be seen before their first session (even after arriving at the office for an initial visit). Many patients have seen me on television or read newspaper articles in which I was quoted after the tragedy of September 11th. Many patients were surprised to discover that I am a Muslim, but the majority did not cease treatment. Since the practice of homosexuality is not permitted in Islam, treating homosexual patients presents a dilemma to the Muslim therapist. A few homosexual patients have ceased treatment with me after discovering that I am Muslim. Those who do not know that I am a Muslim are still in treatment.

When I started my private practice in March 2000, I was the first Muslim psychiatrist in the state of Massachusetts to provide mental health services tailored to Muslim patients. I was not aware of how many practicing Muslim psychiatrists were in the Massachusetts area. Two years later, I came to realize that more than 15 Muslim psychiatrists were practicing in the state, seven of whom were in private, outpatient practice. Muslim patients from other cities who were looking for a Muslim psychiatrist have been referred to me, only to find out later that a Muslim psychiatrist practiced in their own city. Many Muslim patients would travel a long distance to see a Muslim mental health professional. In one case, a Muslim patient came to me from Maryland for a consultation.

Collaboration With Faith Communities

The Muslim community is a communally oriented society (Al-Abdul-Jabbar 2000). The Koran and the prophetic teachings emphasize a collective call to the people ("O People," "O Believers"). They recommend that believers pray in congregations. In addition, the other pillars of Islam are group oriented. In Ramadan, the holy month of fasting, Muslims around the world stop and resume eating at the same time. During the annual pilgrimage to Mecca, more than 2 million Muslims gather for a religious ritual. This communal orientation affects the understanding of mental illnesses and their treatment. The patient may consult several family members, friends, or even the imam of the local mosque before seeing a specialist. These tendencies create a dilemma in dealing with serious mental illnesses such as schizophrenia, and a family may attempt to conceal the illness and limit the patient's interaction with the outside world. Families may feel embarrassment and shame from the mental illness of female members because of the potential effect on prospects for marriage and the family's reputation.

The leader of the local community, religious group, or a mosque is known as its imam. In Muslim countries, where a ministry of religious affairs hires the imams (many times against the will of the people), the role of the imam has lost historic respect. In the West, however, the imam is selected by the administrators of the local Islamic center, and he plays an essential role in the life of the local community. He is usually consulted about various religious, social, and psychological issues. Many imams go to local hospitals to visit the sick. Some major local hospitals have even hired an imam to fulfill the role of chaplain.

Many imams in the United States have little or no background in dealing with psychological issues (Rashed 2000). Some hold false beliefs about mental illnesses. However, since the majority of imams in the United States have at least a university-level education, they are often easy to educate about mental health conditions. I started a local effort in the state of Massachusetts to provide mental health awareness and training to local imams and Muslim leaders. Relationships among us have been positive and constructive, and the religious leaders have generated many referrals. More such concerted efforts on the part of Muslim mental health professionals are needed.

Conclusions

In the United States and other Western countries, considerable misinformation clouds the understanding that the public and mental health professionals have of Islam and of Muslims. Clinicians who treat Muslim patients should familiarize themselves both with the basics of Islam as a religion and with the sociological characteristics of Muslims in their local area. Muslims themselves need to revive and further develop Islamic insights into the psyche so that they can help individuals draw on Islam as a resource in the treatment process. Some of these remedies may stand on their own, while others may complement traditional psychiatric remedies.

References

Al-Abdul-Jabbar J, Al-Issa I: Psychotherapy in Islamic Society, in Al-Junun: Mental Illness in the Islamic World. Edited by Al-Issa I. Madison, CT, International Universities Press, 2000, pp 277–293

Alam A: American Muslims: Community at a Crossroads (Project MAPS: Muslims in American Public Square). April 23, 2002. Available at: http://www.projectmaps. com. Accessed September 20, 2002.

Al-Mabarakpuri SR: The Sealed Nectar, Biography of the Noble Prophet, 1st Edition. Riyadh, Saudi Arabia, Maktaba Dar-us-Salam, 1995

Al-Sanee'a S: Religion and Mental Health. Riyadh, Saudia Arabia, Imam Mohammed Ibn Soud University, 2000

Badri M: Contemplation: An Islamic Psychospiritual Study. Translated by Lu'Lu'a AW. Herndon, VA, International Institute of Islamic Thought, 2000

Council on American-Islamic Relations: The Mosque in America: A National Portrait. April 23, 2001. Available at: http://www.cair-net.org/mosquereport. Accessed September 20, 2002.

El-Kadi A: Health and healing in the Quran. Journal of the Islamic Medical Association of South Africa, March 1989, pp 5–7

El-Kadi A, El-Kadi I: A Multimodality Approach in the Treatment of Drug Addiction. Panama City, FL, Institute of Islamic Medicine for Education and Research, 1997

Erickson CD, al-Timimi NR: Providing mental health services to Arab Americans: recommendations and considerations. Cultur Divers Ethnic Minor Psychol 7:308–327, 2001

Hedayat-diba Z: Psychotherapy with Muslims, in Handbook of Psychotherapy and Religious Diversity. Edited by Richards PS, Bergin AE. Washington, DC, American Psychological Association, 2000, pp 289–313

Husain SA: Religion and mental health from the Muslim perspective, in Handbook of Religion and Mental Heath. Edited by Koenig HG. San Diego, CA, Academic Press, 1998, pp 279–290

Pickthall MM: The Meaning of the Glorious Koran: Text and Explanatory Translation. New York, Mostazafan Foundation of New York, 1984

Rashed D: Islamic Perspectives on Mental Illness and Counseling. September 4, 2000. Available at: http://www.islam-online.net/iol-english/dowalia/news-2000-sep-04/topnews7.asp. Accessed September 25, 2002.

Shehu S: Towards an Islamic Perspective of Developmental Psychology. June 17, 2002. Available at: http://www.islamonline.net/english/Contemporary/2002/05/ Article7.shtml. Accessed September 25, 2002.

Zareek M: Islamic Psychology, 2nd Edition. Damascus, Syria, Dar Al-Maarefah, 1993

CHAPTER 9

Hindus and Buddhists

Nalini V. Juthani, M.D.

Introduction

Hinduism developed in India at least 5,000 years ago, and Buddhism emerged from it in the sixth century B.C. In this chapter, these faiths will be considered together for matters in which their similarity allows; for matters in which they differ, Hinduism will be reviewed first and Buddhism second.

India's indigenous culture grew out of antiquity in two large, advanced cities called Mohanjo-Daro and Harappa. The Greeks, who invaded India under Alexander the Great, designated the inhabitants of the bank of the Indus River as *Indoos*, or Hindus, and their religion, which has no known beginning or human founder, as Hinduism (Burke 1996, pp. 13–35; Feurstein et al. 2001, pp. 45–59). The main source of our knowledge of this era is the Vedas, the earliest surviving Hindu scriptures. Although these texts were passed down orally and were transcribed only during the last millennium, the Sanskrit language and the religion and culture of Vedic India had a profound influence on Europe, Asia, and much of the rest of the world. Large numbers of Hindus, approximately 781 million (Information Please Almanac 2004), now reside throughout Asia, Africa, Europe, and North America. It is estimated that more than 1 million Hindus reside in North America (Information Please Almanac 1998).

The founder of Buddhism was born in the sixth century B.C. with the given name Siddharth. He later came to be known as Gautama Buddha, referring to one who is "enlightened" or "one who has woken to the nature and meaning of life." Gautama Buddha was a prince who was raised by his father, the king of Kapilavastu in Northern India, amidst great luxury and was shielded from exposure to unhappiness, sickness, old age, or death. Before Gautama's birth, his father received a disturbing prophecy that his future son was destined to become a great sovereign or a famous ascetic.

When he was 20 years old, Buddha witnessed on the streets of Kapilavastu an old man, a corpse, a sick man, and a peacefully wandering ascetic. Horrified by the realization that sickness, old age, and death were the ultimate fate of all human beings, he was unable to return to the normal pleasures of his palace. Renouncing this worldly life seemed the only way to escape. For the next 6 years, he was a spiritual seeker who looked for answers to the question of why there was sorrow, birth, old age, and death. He began studying yoga and philosophy with two Hindu ascetics, and, when he did not find what he was seeking, he pursued Hindu rituals of self-mortification. When these rituals did not release him from suffering, he parted ways with Hinduism and instead explored a path of intensive self-scrutiny through contemplation and meditation. After 6 days of intense meditation, he was enlightened. He experienced a profound clarification of his search and of his understanding of human existence, which resulted in a vision of the path to eradicate human suffering. He then became an enlightened religious teacher of this vision. Buddha's teachings arose from the background of Hinduism, but rejected Hindu concepts such as authority and tradition, rituals, speculation, grace, mystery, and a personal God (Finn and Rubin 2000). In part because Hindus had become ritualistic rather than introspective about these concepts, Buddhism did not find broad acceptance in India, but it spread extensively from near Patna in Northern India to neighboring countries such as Tibet and China, and then to Japan and other parts of Asia. Today, there are more then 324 million Buddhists throughout the world (Information Please Almanac 2004), with approximately 2 million in the United States (Information Please Almanac 1998).

Perhaps more than in some other faiths, culture and belief are inevitably intertwined for the Hindu and the Buddhist. Religion both influences and is reinforced by family and social structure, as the following example of the Hindu family illustrates.

The traditional Hindu family comprises three generations living under the same roof. The grandfather, as head of the family, makes final decisions. The family name or honor (*izzat*) has great importance in Hindu culture, and males are valued because they continue the family name. A woman, as a daughter, wife, or mother, is dependent on a man, but she gains power and status when she becomes the mother-in-law of her son's wife, who comes to live in her house. Men control decisions in business settings, and women control decisions in family and household affairs, although to an outsider it would seem that the men are in charge. Children are raised to value interdependence. Arranged marriages are expected. Independence is discouraged and is often perceived as arrogance or disrespect toward the family.

Urbanization, industrialization, and migration increasingly threaten this tightly knit family structure with disintegration. In North America, for example, Hindu women become rapidly independent, and children see themselves as individuals. Hindu men feel the loss of the power and status that they held in the traditional hierarchy.

In traditional Hindu society, social status is based on the caste into which a person is born rather than on an individual's merit. The collective identity that determines an individual's ranking is based on the principles of *dharma* (a sense of duty), *karma* (one's day-to-day actions), and the distribution of labor. Hindus believe that one's karma in a previous life determines whether an individual is reincarnated (born in the next birth) into a higher or lower caste. Brahmins, the highest caste, are considered closest to God and are responsible for preaching and conducting rituals. Next come Kshatriyas, who are protectors and fight wars, and Vaishyas, who are professionals, laborers, farmers, and businessmen. Shudra, the lowest caste, carry out the cleaning jobs and are considered "untouchables." The caste system is still prevalent in rural India, where marriages between members of different castes are frowned on, but its importance in modern urban society is significantly less than in the past.

Professions such as medicine, engineering, and computer science are highly valued in India. Indian immigrants come to the West for educational and occupational reasons rather than to escape religious persecution. The immigrants tend to be educated and of middle or higher socioeconomic class and are often the "cream of the crop" of their families. Since Indians value family integrity, as well as education and hard work, many immigrants carry a burden of guilt about leaving family members behind and feel an unspoken expectation that they will eventually support the extended family.

Core Beliefs and Practices

To understand core beliefs and practices of Hinduism, one needs to know that Hinduism is one of the oldest religions of the world. It absorbed earlier belief systems and their varied rituals and practices, some of which were introduced by invaders. Its earliest scripture (Rig-Veda, one of the Vedas) integrates nature gods with Hindu conceptions of mysticism (Easwaran 1990b). Later, Brahmin priests were entrusted with ancient hymns, rituals, and deities from other lands, including Persia. The scriptures of Hinduism— the Vedas, Upanishads, and Bhagavad Gita—were written and compiled progressively at different times during the eras portrayed in the two major epics of Hinduism, the Mahabharata and the Ramayana. Hinduism is therefore a religion that is both diverse and developmental.

Buddhist beliefs and practices developed in stages as texts were translated into the languages of the host cultures. Buddhism retained an Indian connection but engaged in constructive dialogue with other religions and cultures (including North American) and has often been assimilated according to local conditions. As a result, Buddhism today is not a single unified religion. It exists not only in its two major sects (Theraveda and Mahayana) but in a wide variety of forms. Descriptions of beliefs and practices common to Hindus and Buddhists follow, with comments delineating aspects of these beliefs and practices in which the two faiths differ.

Because the beliefs and practices of Hindus and Buddhists reflect cultural diversity and provide room for freedom of thought, fundamentalism is uncommon. Buddhism is a missionary religion in that its monks and nuns travel far and wide to teach Buddha's doctrines, but these missionaries generally assimilate into the culture of the host country.

Creator

Hindus believe in one creator, whom they recognize by many names such as Brahma, Shiva, and Vishnu. The Upanishads call this supreme reality atman, Brahma, or Self, because it is the ground for everyone's divinity. This informing power holds everything together, creates, destroys, and recreates. Rama, Krishna, and Buddha are considered reincarnated forms of the Creator. As a verse in the Bhagavad Gita (song of the spirit) states, "Whenever righteousness declines and the purpose of life is lost, I manifest myself on earth" (Bhaktivedanta 1994). Hindus, therefore, can choose any deity to worship based on their individual faith (Easwaran 1990b). Although Hinduism is in essence a monotheistic faith, this choice of deities to worship has sometimes led to the notion that it is polytheistic.

Buddhism, on the other hand, holds that there is no such thing as a self and therefore no such thing as a being—only becoming. There is no soul that could survive the death of the body; a human being is simply a bundle of forces or energies that come together transiently. By the same token there is no God, no divine substance or entity, and no Atman (Burke 1996).

Reincarnation

Hindus presuppose that there is a soul that departs from a dying body and is reborn in another body. Buddhists believe that although there is no soul that passes from one body to another, there is a causal continuity. At the end of life, our desires and attachments create a karmic spark that ignites a new round of desires and attachments and with them a potential for reincarnation.

Karma

Hindus believe that all actions of human beings are subject to the law of karma, which states that every event is both a cause and an effect. Therefore, each person is responsible for what happens to him or her ("As you sow, so shall you reap"). Good karma (physical or mental) is rewarded, and sinful karma is punished. It follows that one can take destiny into one's hands and, by personal awareness and effort, change oneself. Since karma is an educative force through which the individual is encouraged to pursue life selflessly in service of the welfare of the whole world, Hindus regard life as a school where one learns, skips a grade, graduates, or is held behind. A person has to go through a cycle of life and death as long as the debt of karma remains (Juthani 1998).

Buddhists also believe in karma. Mahayana Buddhists believe that buddhas, or enlightened beings, are filled with compassion and are reservoirs of good karma, which they can transfer to those who petition them. Through pure compassion, buddhas can also take over the evil karma of others. This concept of transferring karma does not exist in Hinduism.

Dharma

Both Hindus and Buddhists share a mindfulness for dharma, holding slightly different meanings for the word. For Hindus, dharma is a sense of duty to the family, society, and the universe. It is the need to conduct oneself in accord with the essential order of things, which brings integrity and harmony to the universe. Dharma includes rightness, goodness, and purpose, the highest form of which is *ahimsa*, or nonviolence through universal love. When Buddhists, monks included, chant each day, "I take refuge in Buddha, I take refuge in dharma, I take refuge in *sangha* (community)," they are referring respectively to the teachings of Buddha, the cosmic law, and the path toward the realization, or nirvana.

Four Noble Truths

Buddha's teachings about human sufferings are summarized in the Four Noble Truths. The first Noble Truth explains that suffering is caused not only by old age, sickness, and death but by change in every aspect of life, including the personal, relational, environmental, and occupational. The second Noble Truth is that desire, attachment, and craving cause suffering ("All creatures love life. All creatures fear death."). Attachment leads to suffering when the object of attachment is lost. Buddha taught that when selfish desires arise, a series of afflictions such as worry, fear, insecurity, alienation, delusion, infatuation, and illness also arise. The third Noble Truth is that suffering can be eradicated. Extinguishing desire releases one from psychological imprisonment and brings complete awakening, or nirvana. In this state, the oneness of all life is experienced. The fourth Noble Truth shows how to experience enlightenment through right understanding, right aspiration, right speech, right action, right livelihood, right effort, right mindfulness, and right concentration (Finn et al. 2000, p. 321).

Bhakti (Devotion)

Hindus see God everywhere and in everything. In addition to having this conscious awareness of the divine in every aspect of daily routine life, Hindus engage in *puja* (the process of worship or devotion) directed toward the Divine Absolute in the form of gods and goddesses. Rituals designed to facilitate closeness and, ultimately, unity with the Absolute are carried out in groups that meet in the temple, whereas individual idol worship takes place in the home. (It is important to note that it is not the idol but the aspect of the Divine Absolute that is worshipped by the devotees.)

Some Mahayana Buddhists devote themselves to receiving the karmic grace of a buddha, especially while they are going through trying periods. Monks organize devotional events that involve gathering at the temple and use of ritual objects, such as pagodas and statues. Buddhists also celebrate festivals that commemorate events in the life of Buddha such as his birthday and the days on which he achieved enlightenment and nirvana. The focus is on aspects of Buddhist nature, not worship of the statue of Buddha.

Meditation

The Buddhist approach to suffering is to alter one's perception of the world through meditation. When the turbulence of distracting thoughts subsides and the mind becomes still, a deep contentment and happiness naturally arise from within. In monasteries, both devotional and meditational Mahayana Buddhists learn the skills and mental discipline of meditation. Buddhist meditation centers flourish in North America, where converts to Buddhism are increasingly prevalent. American Buddhists may be Catholic Buddhists, Protestant Buddhists, atheist Buddhists, or Jewish Buddhists. They may follow their own Buddhist teacher. The practice of meditation varies widely. For example, Tibetan Buddhists, Theravada Buddhists, and Zen Buddhists each have distinctive meditation practices. Such detail is beyond the scope of this chapter; however, the practice of meditation can produce mental experiences that a Western clinician may consider pathological, and these experiences need to be understood in the context of the patient's spiritual tradition.

Summary

The worldview of a Hindu patient considers that the higher power of God is the source of good. One's desires, thoughts, and actions that are not governed righteously according to dharma are the sources of sinful karma. An individual's attachment to desires and egoism produces emotional states of anger, resentment, shame, guilt, low self-esteem, confusion, and loss of a sense of self. These emotional states produce emotional distress. Buddhists, as well as Hindus, believe that submission, gratitude, forgiveness, self-sacrifice, and self-awareness lead to a capacity for detachment that ultimately leads to nirvana. This state in life can be accomplished by sublimation of desires, an ultimate coping skill.

Clinical Implications

Western clinicians need to appreciate the intertwining of Eastern culture and worldview for several reasons. Hindu patients are often concerned about family honor, stigma, and secrecy. Because denial is common in Hindu society, a clinician must ask direct and specific questions to elicit information about issues such as domestic violence, alcoholism, and incest. Since mind, body, and spirit are believed to be on a continuum, clinicians also need to ask if the patient is using ayurvedic medicines, homeopathic medicines, or any other treatments such as meditation and yoga. Since both Hindus and Buddhists regard suffering as an unavoidable teacher on the path to spirituality, they may be willing to suffer so that they can reach beyond an intellectual understanding of spirituality to experience love. They may try to reconcile themselves by saying that their suffering is the result of their karma, or they may try to compensate for their suffering by actions with good karma in the hope that in their next birth, they will have a better life.

An implication of Hindu and Buddhist beliefs about suffering and of the Hindu traditional family structure is that a Hindu or Buddhist patient is rarely self-referred. He or she has generally exhausted all resources, including alternative medicine, consultation with a primary care doctor, and consultation with a guru (spiritual leader), before seeking psychiatric treatment. Several family members who expect to offer some insight into the patient's problem usually accompany a Hindu or Buddhist patient. There is little concern for confidentiality, and in fact family involvement is usually important for the patient's compliance. The clinician should inquire about the expectations of all family members. Both the patient and the family members are likely to expect that the therapist will behave like a guru by giving advice and being active in therapy. Since they expect treatment to be short and goal oriented, cognitive-behavioral therapy is more readily accepted than long-term insight-oriented psychotherapy.

Cross-generational conflicts within the family are common and are often illustrated by problems in marriages. Arranged Hindu marriages are considered social contracts that link not only a man and woman but their two families. The therapist who encounters marital problems may therefore need to assess the expectations of all parties concerned and listen for cross-generational conflicts. It may be advisable to meet with all family members involved. On the other hand, Western therapists typically encounter Hindu immigrants who moved out of the extended family when they migrated to the United States. These couples and members of nuclear families depend on each other for the physical, emotional, and spiritual support that the extended family would normally provide. Hindus do not consider divorce a desirable option.

> A 35-year-old Hindu Indian physician came for treatment because of conflict he felt about buying a house in the United States instead of sending money back home to buy a larger house and support the day-to-day expenses of his extended family. Although he lived with his nuclear family in the United States, he believed that his dharma (duty) as a son was to be the primary caretaker of his parents and siblings, including helping them achieve a higher socioeconomic status. Tension between his own desires to have his nuclear family live comfortably and to fulfill the unspoken expectations of his extended family led him to feel guilty and depressed. It also led to conflicts with his wife and children, who believed he should be loyal to his nuclear family first.
>
> In the course of therapy, his therapist tried to help him clarify both his situation and the source of his values. The patient described how his mother had told him stories of Rama, the ideal son described in the Ramayana, and how she had instilled in him the value of being an ideal son. He also faced the limitations of his own economic situation in the United States and examined the reasons he was at odds with his wife and children. Empathy and encouragement to sort out his feelings and duties as a Hindu helped him to resolve his guilt and indecisiveness. He eventually continued to provide for unexpected expenses of the extended family but stopped taking care of their day-to-day living expenses.

This case illustrates how stories from the Hindu epics, such as those in the Ramayana and Mahabharata that depict the ideal son who sacrifices himself for the betterment of his extended family, can become ingrained in Hindu families. The following case illustrates involvement of extended family members in the psychiatric treatment of a Hindu patient:

> A 28-year-old Hindu woman was brought to the office by her husband, a cousin, and her aunt. She was a new immigrant to the United States, and she

missed her family in India, cried easily, and had developed depression. To cope, she was spending hours in prayer and ritual in the belief that these actions would bring her peace. Her family had supported her until she began continuing the rituals late into the night, during which time she also called her religious guru in India. Recognizing that her religiosity was extending beyond the norm, her family brought her to see a psychiatrist. They were prepared to educate the clinician about their beliefs and were open to becoming involved in the treatment.

In therapy, the patient described the grief and anxiety she felt in the new and unfamiliar environment of the United States. Her family's support helped her to recognize that while her religious beliefs brought her peace, she had lost control of her behavior. Grieving the loss of the familiarity of her country of origin and the loved ones left behind and acknowledging her feelings of insecurity helped her gradually to make the transition to living in a new land.

The family's input in this case helped the clinician to distinguish between religious and cultural practices and a clinical condition. Their support also helped in the treatment of the patient's pathological grieving and depression.

Intergenerational conflicts between Hindu parents and Westernized Hindu children are common. These conflicts often involve areas of dating, sexuality, and the boundaries between the nuclear and extended family. Traditional Hindu parents value arranged marriages, but this concept is repulsive to youngsters who grow up in the West. In traditional Hindu marriage, a woman marries not only a husband but also his family and moves in with his extended family, whereas Western youngsters want a nuclear family with clear independence from the extended family. The following case provides an example of how a Hindu family addressed these issues in treatment:

Hindu parents brought their 18-year-old daughter for treatment because they were concerned that she was an arrogant, disrespectful, independent "Americanized brat." Born in the United States, the patient had grown up with two sets of values—Hindu values at home and Western values outside of the home. She felt controlled by her traditional parents, who did not allow her to date. She also felt isolated and disconnected from her peers.

Treatment included family and individual sessions. In family therapy, her parents expressed their concerns about teenage pregnancy and sexually transmitted diseases. The patient was able to talk in turn about "needing her space" and wanting her parents to trust her judgment. By emphasizing the Hindu values of interdependence, the therapist encouraged the patient to respect her parents' concerns. The parents were pleased enough by this development to allow her to date if she observed the curfew hours they set. In this case, discussing moral and cultural and religious values with the patient and her parents helped them reach a compromise.

Hindus believe that human beings progress through four stages in their lives. The first stage is the student stage, in which the task is to build character. During the householder stage, one gets married and takes on the responsibility of work, family, and society. Pursuit of worldly success, wealth, fame, and power also take place during this stage. In retirement, one begins gradually to focus on the internal self and to develop further spiritually by giving of oneself to improve the welfare of others and carrying out one's duty toward society. The final stage is called *sannyas*, or the ascetic life. In this stage, one begins to give up attachments and lives a life in which desires and expectations gradually subside. The goal is to become one with the Supreme Reality. Hindus respect old age as part of the third and fourth stages of life. They consider death as a necessary event whereby the old body is shed and the immortal soul enters a new body. As Lord Krishna says in the Bhagavad Gita, "Worn out garments are shed by the body. Worn out bodies are shed by the dweller within the body. New bodies are worn by the dweller like garments" (Bhaktivedanta 1994). The scripture further states, "Not wounded by weapons, [n]ot burned by fire, [n]ot wetted by water, [s]uch is the Atman, [n]ot dried, not wetted, [n]ot burned, not wounded, [s]uch is the innermost element which is everywhere, [c]hangeless and eternal, forever and ever" (Easwaran 1992).

Buddhists believe that when the mind is still, we are lifted out of time into an eternal present—a blissful, utter stillness called *shanti*. There is no past or future, and fear of death disappears.

> A 70-year-old woman was referred by her son-in-law and granddaughter after the patient's 48-year-old daughter, her only child, died suddenly of a brain hemorrhage. The woman had not cried and seemed to be in a deep contemplative mode. She explained that her suffering was predestined and caused by her karma from a previous birth and that she was contemplating how she could detach from her daughter's body, given that her daughter's soul was immortal. She also said that she was planning to go to India to spend some time with her guru, who would guide her in further detachment from her daughter. Recognizing the importance of religious coping for this patient in the final stage of her life, the therapist supported her desire to spend time with her guru. As a Buddhist, the woman might also have coped with death by going to a "monk hoot," or place where monks live. Such settings allow individuals to meditate, examine karma, and determine to do positive deeds. With time, the patient began to give up attachment to her daughter.

Belief in reincarnation and karma and receiving the guidance of a guru or monk are the ways in which a bereaved Buddhist or Hindu normally comes to accept a loss and stop grieving. Western psychiatrists should encourage this process rather than begin exploratory work in dynamic psychotherapy with bereaved Buddhist and Hindu patients. If these means of coping do not prevent depression, the clinician can employ psychological approaches simultaneously.

Variations of Therapeutic Encounters

Even if the therapist and patient both hold a Hindu or Buddhist worldview, the therapist still needs to explore the meaning of the patient's worldview, since patients' concerns may vary depending on their stage of spiritual development. When the therapist holds a Hindu or Buddhist worldview and the patient does not, the therapist should explore the patient's worldview nonjudgmentally and avoid imposing his or her own beliefs on the patient.

When a Western clinician treats a Hindu or Buddhist patient, the following points may be clinically useful:

- Identify the spokesperson for the family and listen to that person carefully.
- Explore patients' immigration history, family caste status, and religious values as part of an extended family history.
- Ask about the family's and the patient's expectations about life in the United States and whether they have been able to realize those expectations.
- Inquire about the patient's and the family's values and whether they have come into conflict in the Western world. If the patient is an adolescent growing up in the Western world, explore how the patient manages or fails to manage two sets of values, one at home and another in Western society. Explore conflicts regarding dating and physical intimacy.
- Remain aware of countertransference issues that may be culturally based in order to maintain an open mind and nonjudgmental stance.

Collaboration With Faith Communities

Buddhist and Hindu patients share a belief system in karma and reincarnation. They manage their problems by consulting with family members, wise men and women in the community, and religious elders or gurus. Like a hospital chaplain or pastoral counselor in a Western tradition, the guru may listen and give advice. The guru may also offer prayers, chant, perform rituals, and guide the patient in meditation. He may advise a Buddhist patient to shave the head, wear monk's clothing, and spend some time in a monastery.

A Western therapist should inquire about the patient's faith community and ask the patient to give consent for the therapist to contact the patient's guru or religious elder. In speaking with the guru, the Western therapist should:

- Listen to the guru's description of any culture- or faith-based interventions that the guru may have initiated.

- Ask questions to clarify and educate him- or herself about specific faith-based interventions.
- Ask the guru how he or she feels about the disciple's consultation with a psychiatric therapist.
- Convey that the therapist and guru have a similar goal of establishing harmony in the mind-body-spirit continuum.
- Avoid conveying that a goal is to relieve the patient from suffering, although this goal may also be a concern of the guru.
- Offer collaboration and an exchange of views. For example, the Buddhist belief system and psychodynamic interpretations may overlap in useful ways.
- Keep symptom relief as the goal, and leave personality restructuring to the patient's self-exploration through his or her faith, with the help of the guru and the faith community.
- Learn about the use of ashrams and monasteries as resources for meditation that are available to Hindus and Buddhists in the local community.

Summary

Hindu and Buddhist worldviews have many implications for collaborative treatment. Since Hindu and Buddhist patients and families rarely accept long-term treatment, growth and character change are more likely to occur through religious and spiritual activities than through psychotherapy. Patients who perceive their therapist as a guru may accept cognitive-behavioral therapy. Therapists can often combine traditional healing ceremonies, yoga, and meditation with Western modalities of treatment. A clinician's approval of such faith-based practices and his or her willingness to collaborate with family members and spiritual leaders are often important in achieving a positive outcome.

References

Bhaktivedanta AC (Swami Prabhupada): Bhagavad Gita: As It Is. Los Angeles, CA, The Bhaktivedanta Book Trust, 1994

Burke TP: The Major Religions: An Introduction With Texts. Cambridge, MA, Blackwell, 1996

Easwaran E: The Dhammapada: Translated for the Modern Reader. Tomales, CA, Nilgiri Press, 1990a

Easwaran E: The Upanishad. Tomales, CA, Nilgiri Press, 1990b

Easwaran E: Dialogue with Death: A Journey Into Consciousness. Tomales, CA, Nilgiri Press, 1992

Feurstein G, Kak S, Frawley D: In Search of the Cradle of Civilization: New Light on Ancient India. Wheaton, IL, Quest Books, 2001

Finn M, Rubin J: Psychotherapy with Buddhists, in Handbook of Psychotherapy and Religious Diversity. Edited by Richards PS, Bergin AE. Washington, DC, American Psychological Association, 2000, pp 317–340

Information Please Almanac: Non-Christian Religious Adherents in the United States (from 1998 Britannica Book of the Year). Available at: http://www.infoplease.com/ipa/A0193644.html. Accessed May 10, 2004.

Information Please Almanac: Top Ten Organized Religions of the World. Available at: http://www.infoplease.com/ipa/A0904108.html. Accessed May 10, 2004.

Juthani NV: Understanding and treating Hindu patients, in Handbook of Religion and Mental Health. Edited by Koenig HG. San Diego, CA, Academic Press, 1998, pp 271–278

CHAPTER 10

Atheists and Agnostics

Syed Atezaz Saeed, M.D.

Richard L. Grant, M.D.

Introduction

Formal worldviews, often termed theistic or atheistic, as well as less formal worldviews, sometimes termed spiritual or agnostic, usually include specific tenets or beliefs that shape experience and influence behavior. A working knowledge of the most commonly encountered worldviews is important not only to help clinicians become more culturally sensitive but also to help them appreciate the potential therapeutic resources and drawbacks that various traditions may offer. However, attempting to write about atheism and agnosticism as worldviews in a manner parallel to specific faith traditions is inherently difficult. As worldviews, these two approaches are defined primarily by their rejection of religion and spirituality as relevant to understanding the human condition. Atheists and agnostics typically do not see their views as "faith-based." They do hold that the divergent epistemologies of religion or spirituality and atheism or agnosticism lead to different conclusions about answers to *proximate* questions (How do unhealthy, maladaptive, or symptomatic responses in mental and bodily disorders originate?) and *ultimate* questions (How did we and the universe come to exist? What is our "purpose" in life? What is our fate after death?).

In general, before taking into account their patients' worldviews, atheist and agnostic clinicians do not consider ultimate questions relevant for the delivery of health care services. On the other hand, answers to proximate questions become very relevant. Given some of these fundamental epistemological differences, the goal of this chapter is to identify core features of atheism and agnosticism and discuss the implications of these worldviews in dealing with common clinical issues. The chapter will also consider the effects on the process of psychotherapy of the differing worldviews of patient and therapist.

Terms like atheism and agnosticism have multiple meanings, and neither is a religion or arguably a complete ethical system. *Atheism* is the belief that no deity or deities exists. The American Atheists (2002) define an atheist to be a person who "does not believe in a god or gods, or other supernatural entities." *Agnosticism* is a belief or process of thinking (Eller 2004) that holds we cannot prove either the existence or the nonexistence of a deity or deities or supernatural forces. Many agnostics believe that, given the current state of science and technology, we cannot know anything about a deity or deities presently, but that this circumstance could possibly change in the future.

Atheism

The Encyclopedia Britannica Online (2002) offers perhaps one of the most comprehensive definitions of atheism: "the denial of metaphysical beliefs in God or spiritual beings." By this definition, atheism is more than just a rejection of the core concepts of Judeo-Christianity and Islam—it includes rejection of both anthropomorphic and nonanthropomorphic gods. This definition also includes rejection of the concept of God portrayed by some contemporary thinkers, such as new-age mystics who suggest that God is just another name for love or moral ideals. What is crucial in this definition is not just the idea that an atheist rejects the existence of God but, more importantly, rejects *a belief in God*.

A study of Western thought reveals that atheism has been rooted in many philosophical systems. The philosophic origins of atheism can be traced back to the works of Plato, Democritus, and Epicurus. In the sixteenth century, Machiavelli asserted the independence of politics from religion and in so doing contributed to atheism in the political arena. In the eighteenth century, atheism can be seen in the works of the French Encyclopedists. Both David Hume and Immanuel Kant, although neither one was an atheist, contributed to atheism by arguing against the traditional proofs for the existence of God.

One of the most important nineteenth-century atheists was Ludwig Feuerbach (1841/1989), who argued that God was a projection of man's ideals. In his view, the denial of God would affirm man's freedom and liberate him for self-realization. Drawing on Feuerbach's thesis, Karl Marx further held that religion reflected socioeconomic order and diminished the independent strivings of individuals (Marx and Engels 1964). At about the same time period Marx was refining his concepts of atheism rooted in socioeconomic theory, Charles Darwin was developing a scientific theory of natural selection. Darwin's theory, although never explicitly stated, challenged the very core concept of the Creator-God. In his psychoanalytic theory, Sigmund Freud argued that belief in God represented a regressive childlike state in which God was the projected image of a comforting father figure.

Many twentieth century atheists are existentialists, as exemplified by the works of Friedrich Nietzsche, Jean-Paul Sartre, Albert Camus, and others. Atheistic existentialists maintain that true human freedom requires denial of God because God's existence takes free ethical choice away from human beings and hence interferes with the freedom to create their own values. In other words, denial of God is seen as freedom for humanity to fulfill itself and find its own real meaning. It should be noted that some existentialist thinkers, such as Søren Kierkegaard, have held a religious worldview, espousing freedom in the context of a created moral order.

Further contributions to atheism came from the school of empiricist epistemology and the philosophical movement referred to as logical positivism. David Hume, Thomas Huxley, John Stuart Mill, and many others contributed to empiricist epistemology. This view posits that meaningful knowledge comes from experience and observation. Logical positivism holds that the discussions concerning the existence or nonexistence of God are meaningless and that discussing an unverifiable God is similarly fruitless.

In the mental health field, religion has been viewed in various ways, including from an atheistic perspective. For example, Freud viewed it as an illusion, an obsession, and a fulfillment of infantile wishes; Carl Jung saw it as an archetype; William James described it as an intensely personal experience; B.F. Skinner described it as a result of operant conditioning; Abraham Maslow saw it as a quest for humankind's higher nature; and Viktor Frankl described it as a search for ultimate meaning. Albert Ellis, one of the most outspoken atheist mental health professionals, wrote, "I am inclined to reverse Voltaire's famous dictum and to say that, from a mental health standpoint, if there was a God it would be necessary to uninvent Him" (Ellis 1962, p. 142).

Religious beliefs influence the lives of people with faith in many different ways. Although religious concepts can be used to restructure and improve a patient's psychological problems, sometimes religious beliefs and practices can also be at the root of or can exacerbate these problems (Barshinger and LaRowe 1985; Beck 1985; Berry 1985; Bixler 1985; Edkins 1985; Gibson 1985; Malony 1985).

Agnosticism

Agnosticism refers to the doctrine that we cannot know of the existence of anything beyond the phenomena of our experience. In general, agnosticism leaves open the question of whether God exists. Huxley, a British biologist who popularized philosophical agnosticism, is credited for coining the term *agnostic* in 1869.

Although it may appear that agnosticism is no more than the suspension of judgment on ultimate questions because of insufficient evidence, the essence of agnosticism is not a declaration of total ignorance. Agnosticism is a method, rather than a creed, that emphasizes that humankind must follow reason to its fullest extent and accept the limits of knowledge. This principle was perhaps best illustrated by W. K. Clifford, the British mathematician and philosopher of science, in an essay on "The Ethics of Belief" (1876), in which he wrote: "It is wrong always, everywhere, and for anyone, to believe anything upon insufficient evidence" (Burger 2001).

The origins of agnosticism can be traced back to the Sophists and to Socrates in the fifth century B.C. Hume, perhaps the most important source of agnostic ideas, started from the general empiricist claim that matters of fact and real existence could not be known a priori (prior to and apart from experience). He further argued that one could not know a priori that any thing was or was not the cause of any other thing. These reflections challenged all of the classical arguments for the existence of God with the exception of the argument from design (i.e., the order and structure of the universe is such that there must be a designer for it). In his later works, Hume addressed the design argument by stating that whatever order we recognized should be attributed to the universe itself and not to any postulated outside cause. Hume's position, like Kant's, was that knowledge in this area is practically impossible.

Unlike atheism, agnosticism may have religious forms. However, there are limits to how far one can go in combining religious ideology with agnosticism. A calculated commitment to a faith that includes features of agnosticism is exemplified by the Wager Argument, articulated by Blaise Pascal in the seventeenth century. He suggested that the only sane bet was Roman Catholicism, for one had only a short life to lose if God did not exist, yet eternity to gain if God did exist. Agnosticism is also incompatible with Fideism, the thesis that truth in religion is accessible only to faith. Agnostics cannot accept a faith without some substantiating evidence. The fact that there are limitations to human knowledge is not enough to sustain religious agnosticism. In summary, agnostics affirm that they do not, or cannot, know whether God exists. Unlike atheists, agnostics do not make the definitive statement of saying that God does not, or cannot, exist. Like atheists, they reject the validity of "revealed truths."

There are difficulties in accurately assessing the prevalence of nonbelievers, either atheists or agnostics, in the general population. Yet, a consensus emerges from several different sources. The American Religious Identification Study (ARIS), a large-scale study of more than 50,000 American adults, indicated that the number of Americans who do not identify with any particular religion is growing (Kosmin and Mayer 2001). In 1990, for instance, 90% of adults considered themselves part of a faith-based group; in 2001 that figure dropped to 81%. Not identifying with any religion, however, does not necessarily mean that the other 19% were agnostics or atheists. In 1990, 14.3 million United States adults, or roughly 8%, identified with the nonbeliever category, and in 2001 the nonbeliever population had grown to 29.4 million, roughly 14.1% of the American community. This study estimated that there are 991,000 agnostics in the United States, 0.5% of the total population. The ARIS team noted that the 1990 figure "may be downwardly biased due to a slight change in the wording of the key survey question in 2001. In seeking a more accurate measure of identification, the clause 'if any' was added this year to the question, 'What religion do you identify with?'" (Kosmin and Mayer 2001).

According to the Information Please Almanac (1998), 0.3% of total United States population is atheist and another 8.8% is "nonreligious," but the almanac does not provide a breakdown for the "nonreligious" group.

Finally, according to a study by the Barna Research Group (1999), "roughly 7% of the adult population—approximately 14 million people—described themselves as atheistic or agnostic. This means that America has more atheists and agnostics than Mormons (by a 3 to 1 margin), Jews (by a 4 to 1 margin) or Muslims (by a 14 to 1 margin)." The researchers further found that atheists and agnostics were dominated by whites (71%), men (64%), adults under age 35 years (51%), and residents of the Northeast and West (56%). These findings suggest that atheism and agnosticism are worldviews with which a significant portion of the population identifies, likely in the range of 8% to 14% of the population.

Core Beliefs and Practices

Atheism and agnosticism are not types of "religion," and, although no specific belief systems are specified by these worldviews, both rest on a materialistic, philosophical foundation. Atheists and agnostics believe only what is scientifically verifiable. Unlike religious creeds, the scientific method provides them with a constantly growing body of knowledge about the universe. While the growth in knowledge provides answers to many questions, it also raises new questions. Atheists and agnostics believe that their hold on "truth" is always partial and subject to change as new findings emerge. Within this materialistic-scientific approach to the universe around them, atheists and agnostics enjoy considerable freedom of thought and diversity.

It is in dealing with the *ultimate* questions (such as, How did we and the universe come to exist? What is our "purpose" in life? What is our fate after death?) that major epistemological differences between atheism-agnosticism and faith-based worldviews become obvious. For example, the belief that there is no God means that there is no one to answer prayer, that there is no chance for life after death, and that people must face the consequences of their acts without reference to a religious or spiritual source of morality. Several resources exist for further understanding of atheism and agnosticism (Burger 2001; Dictionary of the History of Ideas 1977; Huxley 1992; Robertson 1972).

Faith-based worldviews at times frame illnesses, disorders, or disordered behavior as a moral failure. By contrast, such difficulties are not viewed by nonreligious worldviews as due to a moral failure but as a malfunction. Atheists and agnostics do not believe in a life after death but value life on earth and the attempt to improve it. The materialistic philosophy of atheism relies on the power of knowledge and the ability of humankind to comprehend the secrets of nature and to create a social system based on reason and justice. In essence, the "faith" a materialist has is in humankind and its ability to transform the world by its own efforts. In health, the fundamental nature of this philosophy is optimistic and life offering, and this philosophy considers the struggle for progress as a moral obligation. It is out of this moral obligation that noble ideals emerge to inspire creativity, discovery, and social justice.

Many agnostics and atheists have a negative attitude toward religions, primarily from the harm done in the name of religion, as well as from the stigma and discrimination of being in a nonreligious minority. Agnostics and atheists believe that distortions about health are promulgated by religious worldviews. Many feel that reliance on a deity on one hand interferes with one's ability to interact with fellow human beings and on the other hand is likely to reduce our motivation to solve our own problems, leading us to ignore many clear sources of health difficulties and their effective remediation. Many atheists and agnostics think that traditional beliefs are often supported by fear of eternal punishment after death and by fear of retaliation by an angry and vengeful God during this lifetime. They think that to live in such fear is unhealthy. In addition, such religious influences promote the idea that perfectly natural feelings, such as anger, lust, pride, and wanting things, are evil and sinful. This idea leads to feelings of guilt and to unnecessary chronic stress and its attendant deleterious effect on the brain and body. This thinking may also lead to unnecessary self-denigration.

Clinical Implications

Atheists and agnostics are more likely to view mental illness as our field views it, just like any other medical condition. They are also more likely to accept treatment. It is less likely that atheists and agnostics would hold a negative bias against mental disorders that would interfere with their scientific view of mental disorders and, therefore, their acceptance of treatment. However, stigma is not entirely a function of belief or religiosity, and atheists and agnostics may not be without bias against mental disorders and their treatment.

The atheistic therapist sees psychopathology in a materialistic way as the expression of brain malfunction due to the combined interaction of genetics and life experience of an individual. Regardless of the variety of explanations offered by the patient for the presence of symptoms, such as a moral failing, the atheistic clinician's treatment recommendations will be pragmatically driven by the symptoms and evidence-based knowledge of what to do about them. Some religious patients continue to see their problems as related to moral failings, and this view presents a challenge to the atheistic therapist who works with religious patients.

The following cases illustrate how a materialistic psychiatrist worked with the religious worldviews of disparate patients to accomplish desired changes in their circumstances or disordered behavior. In no instance were the patient's religious views challenged or a focus of change.

The 19-year-old son of a staunchly conservative religious family was using multiple illicit drugs, including alcohol and cocaine, was living at home, and was not working. Prayer and pastoral counseling were ineffective. Standard substance abuse treatment likewise led to no change in his behavior. The psychiatrist diagnosed bipolar II disorder and attention-deficit/hyperactivity disorder. Pharmacological treatment along with considerable family work led to his stopping the illicit drugs and to stabilization of his life. He was not religious, but his parents attributed his recovery to their and their friends' prayers.

A 35-year-old, married white woman suffered frequent and significant physical abuse from her husband. He told her she was disobedient to the tenets of their religion for her misbehavior in not following his directions for how she should keep the house, treat the children, and engage in other domestic activities. Her sexual disinterest was also a major difficulty. The couple had conferences with their minister in which the husband's role definition was reinforced, but the minister counseled against physical abuse. In therapy with the psychiatrist, the woman opposed redefining her role from the religious perspective. Divorce was initially out of the question, but in therapy she reframed the abuse as a violation of her basic rights within her religion, and she decided to divorce when her husband refused, after a significant span of time, to change his behavior. Her religious faith remained unchanged.

A 45-year-old, white married man worked as a Catholic family life instructor with his wife. The man had had intimations of a gay orientation when he almost went into the seminary as a late teen. A year before he was seen by the psychiatrist, he had a single homosexual encounter with a friend. This experience led to his becoming convinced that he wished to divorce his wife and be in a committed homosexual relationship. At the same time, the patient was incensed when his wife helped their youngest daughter, age 16, to get birth control pills. The daughter was rebellious and had attention-deficit/hyperactivity disorder and oppositional defiant disorder. When confronted with the discrepancy between his attitude toward contraception and being gay, he was clear. The prohibition against contraception and sex outside of marriage were basic to his religion. His daughter should not have the pill. When asked how he justified his homosexuality, given the Pope's recent statements, he said, "Well, the Pope and the church are wrong about that." Now divorced, he lives with a committed partner and runs an AIDS support program in the community. He regularly attends church.

A white man in his mid-40s who was an Apostolic Christian and a white-collar worker had been twice "shunned" by his church for unfaithfulness and zoophilia. His zoophilia-related behavior was not stopped by this shunning, which was a religion-sanctioned form of "treatment." The problems were viewed as a moral failing, but prayer and punishment were ineffective. Referred to a psychiatrist who was a certified sex specialist, he and his wife were seen together and separately. Both agreed to a course of Depo-Provera (medroxyprogesterone acetate) that, within 3 weeks, effectively eliminated his sexual obsession without affecting his sexual behavior with his wife. He declared he had not realized that he had been preoccupied with sexual thoughts "24–7" until they were suppressed.

Suffering patients commonly reexamine their beliefs and other assumptions about life. Religious patients often struggle with the idea of whether God still cares about them or has caused their suffering because they have failed morally. Atheist patients may also search for the meaning of suffering in their lives but reject the answers offered by traditional religions (Peteet 2001).

Dying is a difficult and unpleasant process for most. How we prepare ourselves for this inevitable event varies depending on many factors, such as our convictions, our accomplishments, and our unfinished aspirations, to name just a few. As death approaches, atheists must be at peace with their conviction that they are approaching the natural, anticipated end of a journey and that there is no afterlife. How they face death and dying depends on how successfully they have come to terms with this position, not just as an intellectual exercise but as a true conviction. Death and dying is often an area of fruitful clinical exploration.

Other issues associated with death and dying may be significant for atheist and agnostic patients. One issue is how they have handled the fear of death. As Timothy Leary described it:

... most human beings are taught to face death, like life, as victims—helpless, fearful, resigned. We're schooled and counseled—programmed to act
out a life of scripts based on our worst tendencies toward fear and self-doubt.
Throughout history "fear of dying" has been used by priests, police, politi-
cians, and physicians to undermine individualistic thinking, to increase our
dependence on authority and to glorify victimization. (Leary and Sirius
1997, p. 110)

Atheists and agnostics may also have concerns, perhaps even ambivalence,
regarding what happens to their bodies after they die. Religions are involved
in nearly every aspect of death and dying, and the extent to which the religion may be involved is a decision that is usually made by family members
and significant others. Atheists' nonbeliefs are often superseded by the beliefs of these significant others. Atheists need to successfully resolve these issues. Much of the resolution may be a matter of the atheist's taking a few
practical steps, such as making his or her wishes clear and insisting on arrangements after death that are consistent with his or her beliefs and conducted without religious involvement. From a clinical standpoint, making
such arrangements may also require exploration and processing.

The son and guardian of a 99-year-old mother who died within 3 days after
hospitalization for a fractured femur struggled with how to ensure respect for
her lifelong agnosticism. She had sufficient Alzheimer's disease to warrant
her spending her last 4 years in a care center. Staff there would sometimes
give her religious materials despite requests for that not to happen. She was
friendly and would joke and smile about being given these materials, but her
son had difficulty keeping her from being visited by pastoral counselors. She
had accepted her inevitable death and had said about 15 years ago, "I didn't
know it was going to last this long."

Another important life-spectrum issue is the raising and nurturing of
children. It has been argued that religious belief is necessary for instilling
values and raising children with high moral standards, because morality
does not make sense and life is meaningless without belief in God. Atheists
and agnostics think that even if there is no purpose to life that there are purposes in life. What people care about and want to do can remain perfectly
intact even in a world without God. Atheists and agnostics believe that love,
honesty, friendship, compassion, and solidarity are human goods even in a
godless world. The findings of the Barna Research Group (1999) showed
that atheist and agnostic groups exhibited strong "family values" and had
some of the lowest (if not the lowest) divorce rates, compared to any other
religious group.

Variations of Therapeutic Encounters

Few data exist to guide the behavior of practitioners in this area. Searches in the psychological, psychiatric, and medical literature combining "atheist, agnostic, and psychotherapy" in varying forms and combinations yielded a paucity of literature, in contrast to the burgeoning number of articles found with terms such as "faith-based" or "spirituality" combined with "psychotherapy." Some psychotherapeutic literature addresses existential aloneness and meaninglessness, yet falls short of discussing frank atheism (Yalom 1980). Certainly, the literature is silent on the effect an atheistic or agnostic therapist may have on the therapeutic encounter. Propositions about the role of nonreligious therapists and patients in psychotherapy are very infrequent and rarely evidence based. Many factors may account for this lack of literature, but the preponderance of writers and researchers interested in these issues consider themselves religious, which introduces the possibility of bias, however unintended, into their studies and publications.

However, one can envision simplistically a four-celled matrix of therapists and people with mental disorders that would consist of religious and nonreligious therapists and religious and nonreligious potential patients. Because those people who strongly view their disorders as originating from sinfulness or other religiously based causes may not seek or may reject medical or psychological interventions, these people may not appear in the matrix. Of the rest (i.e., people who do seek out psychological assistance for mental disorders), some will hold a mixture of religious, social, psychological, and biological causative explanations. Others will hold clearly to biological origins for their symptoms and maladaptive behaviors.

Likewise, psychotherapists hold a continuum of views about causation of disorders. How, then, should an almost random pairing of seeker and helper best function for the ultimate goal of cure, control of symptoms, or stemming of deterioration? The "goodness of fit" concept maximizes the possibility of matching the therapist's and patient's worldviews, which may potentially minimize conflicts about causation and approach to treatment. Whether matched combinations of nonreligious therapist and patient or religious therapist and patient are equally effective is for research to determine. The two nonmatched combinations may or may not have differences about causation and treatment. As previous research on psychotherapy suggested, a therapist and patient who do not like one another generally engage in a short, unsuccessful course of psychotherapy (Parloff et al. 1978). Very discrepant worldviews probably have the same influence. Empirical evidence indicates that the underutilization of mental health services by individuals with strong religious worldviews occurs, in part, because of concern that their belief system will be disregarded or, worse, pathologized (Larson et al.

1984, 1989; Shafranske and Malony 1990). No empirical data that directly address this issue from an atheistic or agnostic perspective were found. Thus research directly addressing this question would be necessary to provide a definite answer. However, one could make an inferential leap and hypothesize that these considerations might not be relevant for nonbelievers.

Yet, a stigma remains with "coming out" as an atheist or agnostic (Silverman 2002). Although most atheist or agnostic mental health consumers likely do not realize it, such "coming out" to a therapist should not necessarily be cause for uncertainty or concern about being judged—studies indicate that mental health professionals are less religiously inclined than the national norm. Bergin and Jensen, cited in a report of the National Institute for Healthcare Research (2002), found that 28% of the clinical psychologists and 21% of the psychiatrists responding to their national survey endorsed atheism or agnosticism as their religious preference, compared to 6% in the general population. Further, mental health professionals adhering to full ethical principles will be equally accepting of any worldview held by a patient, regardless of their own worldview.

As a result, the role a patient's worldview plays in his or her life is essential for the therapist to know in collaboratively designing the treatment. Every patient should expect multimodal biopsychosocial treatment. Therapists may choose, if deemed necessary, to inform patients with a worldview discrepant from their own about significant differences that may arise between the therapist's limits and the patient's needs. Referrals to a psychopharmacologist or a spiritual guide are equally appropriate if the therapist is not expert in those modalities. For example, one of us (R.L.G.) treated a Mexican-American patient in Colorado with systems-oriented conjoint work, cognitive-behavioral therapy and medications for depression, and a referral to a *curandera,* a type of shaman or healer.

Clinicians who decide to approach religious or spiritual problems within the psychotherapeutic context can do so at various levels (Peteet 1994). Working at the level of greatest involvement (i.e., addressing the spiritual problem directly within the framework of treatment through use of a shared religious or spiritual orientation), is fraught with the greatest risk of mistakes because of countertransference or shared blind spots. In the same way that a religious therapist and religious patient might collude to avoid facing a fear of dying, an atheistic therapist might collude with an atheistic patient to assume that the patient's rejection of his or her family's faith is simply rational and without psychological significance.

Patients who know that their therapist is an atheist may be hesitant to bring up issues related to their religious beliefs for fear of being judged by a nonbeliever therapist. An atheist or agnostic therapist is more likely to approach this area solely with a scientific view and may attribute a religiously based experience to psychopathology. Such patients can also evoke particular countertransference responses because of the nature of their conflicts (Peteet 1981).

It would be imprudent for an atheist or agnostic therapist to deny or ignore the presence of religious beliefs in the life of a patient for whom these beliefs are an important matter, but religious patients may also sometimes benefit from an alternative perspective. The atheist or agnostic therapist can approach the area of religious belief just as he or she would approach any other ethical dilemma that arises in treatment and that typically reflects the tension between the need to stimulate the patient to think independently and the need for the patient to provide informed consent. Even without a religious faith, atheist and agnostic therapists can be more effective when working with religious patients by familiarizing themselves with religious beliefs and practices of such patients (Warnock 1989). Therapists may sometimes be able to help patients with differing worldviews to integrate their suffering through reframing, accepting the view that the disorder is a punishment, and offering parallel, alternative explanations.

When a patient is an atheist or agnostic and knows that the therapist is not, the patient may fear, at least initially, that the therapist may try to influence his or her beliefs, despite the fact that the mental health profession has a long history of therapists not forcing their values and beliefs on the client and also has ethical codes that reinforce this position. Of course, an atheist or agnostic patient will be less likely to accept treatment from a pastoral counselor, Christian therapist, or a practitioner who uses other religiously based therapeutic approaches. An atheist or agnostic patient who knowingly chooses such a therapist may be interested in reevaluating his or her beliefs.

Atheism and agnosticism have in common a materialistic philosophical foundation. This philosophy regards the world as it actually is and views it in context of the data provided by science and social experience. Materialism is a logical outcome of scientific knowledge gained over the centuries. Persons who accept materialism hold that nothing exists but natural phenomena and that there are no supernatural forces or entities. It is this materialistic philosophy that makes atheism and agnosticism consistent with a scientific approach. Given this philosophy and in the absence of contrary empirical evidence, one can speculate that atheists and agnostics would be more likely to endorse a data-driven approach to mental health treatment and thus to support evidence-based practice, the current major trend in the mental health field.

Collaboration With Faith Communities

Although at first guess one might suppose less collaboration between atheistic and agnostic mental health professionals with faith communities, in some cases it is particularly important for the atheist or agnostic mental health professional to develop a collaborative relationship with a patient's religious leader. For example, in the treatment of scrupulosity as seen in obsessive-compulsive disorder (OCD), it may be particularly helpful, after the therapist and patient have created an exposure hierarchy (which most certainly will involve exposure to some form of religious obsession, be it a thought, image, or impulse), for the patient to seek the counsel of his or her religious leader to receive the leader's approval to engage in the exposure sessions (Ciarrocchi 1995). This step may be difficult because the religious leader may not have an understanding of OCD, but receiving the approval of the religious leader may facilitate the exposure and ritual prevention treatment. Similarly, religious leaders should recognize that a follower's consistent questioning of religious ideas may not indicate interest in (or skepticism about) theological matters but instead may represent obsessive rumination. Collaboration between mental health providers and religious leaders is also likely to be particularly useful in the treatment of patients who experience excessive thoughts of guilt or of being punished. Although these thoughts may at times seem to have a religious genesis, they may, in fact, be instances of the depressive ruminations that can accompany a major depressive episode. In this situation, input from a religious leader may help correct the follower's distorted thinking.

Atheists and agnostics do not have formal faith communities, and mental health professionals typically will not be able to utilize this type of resource for diagnostic or treatment purposes. However, this lack of a faith community should not prevent a therapist from inquiring whether an atheist patient has informal group or communal support from others who share his or her worldview.

In summary, in some instances, it may be in the best interest of a patient for a mental health professional to consult and collaborate with a religious leader. Likewise, there are times when a religious leader should recognize that a follower with excessive religious questioning has mental health difficulties and should refer the person to a mental health professional. Although this collaboration may be difficult because of the differing worldviews, if both "sides" keep in mind that the collaborative effort is in the best interest of the patient and religious follower, a successful collaboration is more likely to result.

References

American Atheists: Visitors' Center: Introduction. Parsippany, NJ, American Atheists, 2002. Available at: http://www.atheists.org/visitors.center/. Accessed October 17, 2002.

Barna Research Group: Atheists and agnostics infiltrating Christian churches. Ventura, CA, Barna Research Group, 1999

Barshinger C, LaRowe L: A developmental pacing of theology in therapeutic process. Journal of Psychology and Christianity 4:62–64, 1985

Beck JR: Post-conversion symptom regression. Journal of Psychology and Christianity 4:19–21, 1985

Berry CM: Dependent personality disorder: case conference. Journal of Psychology and Christianity 4:42–47, 1985

Bixler WG: A terrible, swift sword: Christ imagery in therapy. Journal of Psychology and Christianity 4:37–41, 1985

Burger AJ (ed): The Ethics of Belief: Essays by William Kingdom Clifford, William James, AJ Burger. Roseville, CA, Dry Bones Press, 2001

Ciarrocchi JW: The Doubting Disease: Help for Scrupulosity and Religious Compulsions. Mahwah, NJ, Paulist Press, 1995

Dictionary of the History of Ideas. New York, Charles Scribner's Sons, 1973

Edkins W: Psychoanalysis and religious experience. Journal of Psychology and Christianity 4:86–90, 1985

Eller D: Agnosticism: the basis for atheism, not an alternative to it. American Atheist, Winter 2003–2004, p 37. Available at: http://www.americanatheist.org/win03-04/T1/eller.html. Accessed June 3, 2004.

Ellis A: Reason and emotion in psychotherapy. Secaucus, NJ, Lyle Stuart, 1962

Encyclopedia Britannica Online: Agnosticism. Available at: http://www.britannica.com. Search by word or select topic from alphabetical list. Accessed October 17, 2002.

Encyclopedia Britannica Online: Atheism. Available at: http://www.britannica.com. Search by word or select topic from alphabetical list. Accessed October 17, 2002.

Feuerbach L: The Essence of Christianity (1841). Translated by Eliot G. Amherst, NY, Prometheus Books, 1989

Gibson DL: Doubting Thomas, the obsessive. Journal of Psychology and Christianity 4:34–36, 1985

Kosmin BA, Mayer E: American Religious Identification Survey. New York, Graduate Center of the City University of New York, 2001. Available at: http://www.gc.cuny.edu/studies/aris_index.htm. Accessed July 31, 2002.

Huxley TH: Agnosticism and Christianity, and Other Essays. Amherst, NY, Prometheus Books, 1992

Information Please Almanac: Non-Christian Religious Adherents in the United States (from Britannica Book of the Year), 1998. Available at: http://www.infoplease.com/ipa/A0193644.html. Accessed October 17, 2002.

Larson DB, Pattison EM, Blazer DG, et al: Systematic analysis of research on religious variables in four major psychiatric journals, 1978–1982. Am J Psychiatry 143:329–334, 1984

Larson DB, Donahue M, Lyons J, et al: Religious affiliations in mental health research samples as compared with national samples. J Nerv Ment Dis 177:109–111, 1989

Leary TF, Sirius RU: Design for Dying. New York, Harper-Edge, 1997

Malony HN: A tardy pilgrim. Journal of Psychology and Christianity 4:5–8, 1985

Marx K, Engels F: On Religion. New York, Oxford University Press, 1964

National Institute for Healthcare Research: The Forgotten Factor, Module 1: Charting the Religious Commitment Gap. Rockville, MD, National Institute for Healthcare Research, 2002. Available at: http://www.leaderu.com/orgs/nihr/docs/ff/module1.html. Accessed October 17, 2002.

Parloff MB, Waskow IE, Wolfe BE: Research on therapist variables in relation to process and outcome, in Handbook of Psychotherapy and Behavior Change: An Empirical Analysis, 2nd Edition. Edited by Garfield SL, Bergin A. New York, John Wiley & Sons, 1978

Peteet JR: Issues in the treatment of religious patients. Am J Psychother 35:559–564, 1981

Peteet JR: Approaching spiritual problems in psychotherapy: a conceptual framework. J Psychother Pract Research 3:237–245, 1994

Peteet JR: Putting suffering into perspective: implications of the patient's worldview. J Psychother Pract Res 10:187–192, 2001

Robertson JM: A Short History of Freethought, Ancient and Modern. New York, Arno Press, 1972

Shafranske EP, Malony HN: Clinical psychologists' religious and spiritual orientations and their practice of psychotherapy. Psychotherapy 27:72–78, 1990

Silverman D: Coming out—Atheism: The Other Closet. Parsippany, NJ, American Atheists, 2002. Available at: http://www.atheists.org/comingout/othercloset.html. Accessed October 17, 2002.

Warnock SDM: Rational-emotive therapy and the Christian client. Journal of Rational-Emotive and Cognitive-Behavioral Therapy 7:263–274, 1989

Yalom I: Existential Psychotherapy. New York, Basic Books, 1980

PART IV

Worldview and Culture

CHAPTER 11

Worldview in Global Perspective

Samuel B. Thielman, M.D., Ph.D.

Although the literature on worldview in psychiatry is relatively sparse, there is a longstanding, natural connection between anthropology and psychiatry. Writing on the relationship between culture and mental health has called considerable attention to the importance of worldview in properly understanding and treating mental disorders.

Culture is a broadly inclusive term used to describe the shared beliefs and behaviors of a group of people. It is often seen as constantly changing. *Worldview*, on the other hand, is the philosophical outlook that a person, knowingly or not, utilizes to organize his or her activities. It is much more a function of an individual self. Hence culture is more the province of anthropology, and worldview, that of philosophy. Psychiatric clinicians need to consider both worldview and culture; culture shapes worldview and worldview affects an individual's ability to accept the treatments, especially the psychotherapeutic treatments, that are offered. This consideration of worldview and culture is increasingly important as clinicians treat ever larger groups of people—often people living in or coming from non-Western contexts—affected by war, terrorism, and natural disasters. Much of the psychiatric literature on culture has focused on nuances of cultures within North America and Western Europe. Yet the range of worldviews held by individuals across the world is far greater than what an American or European psychiatrist normally sees in his or her practice. A growing literature now addresses cultural aspects of treating the very large and diverse populations of Africa; the Middle East; South, Central, East, and Southeast Asia; and Central and South America.

As Western culture extends further into the various traditional cultures of the world, it brings with it secular models of mental health treatment. These models take hold not only among populations affected by catastrophe but also among more affluent, urbanized populations. The result is increasing engagement between traditional worldviews and the secular worldview of the West. Sometimes the outcome is positive, sometimes negative. Often, the outcome is unexpected. Relief organizations can expend substantial resources on Western psychotherapies for affected populations with an uncertain likelihood that these interventions will have an effect (Summerfield 1999), which brings into high relief the importance of worldview in mental health care delivery. In this chapter, I provide a brief historical review and then consider contemporary clinical implications of this challenge using examples drawn from the African context.

Historical Background

One of the first psychiatric authors to discuss the role of worldview in psychiatric treatment, particularly as it related to religion, was the prominent German psychiatrist Wilhelm Griesinger (1817–1869). At the time he wrote, German psychiatry had been shaped not only by developments in pathophysiology but also by the German romantic movement, which placed a strong emphasis on the role of spirituality in mental well-being (Ackernecht 1968). In fact, some German psychiatrists of the early nineteenth century viewed mental illness as being rooted in spiritual disorder and attributed madness to sinfulness, viewing religion as a principal remedy. Since Germany had large Catholic, Protestant, and Jewish populations, Griesinger grappled with how to address the treatment of mental illness in patients with diverging religious points of view. He cautioned against religious instruction as an attempt to cure patients, but he also noted that for patients who were religiously inclined, religious services were often beneficial. He also entertained the idea that psychiatry could be developed along lines consistent with Catholic, Protestant, and Jewish religious thought. He wrote,

> Several medical psychologists would have the whole treatment of the insane to be specifically Christian. But Jews also require the aid of the alienist and his science and there is no abstract, only a confessional Christianity. Therefore there would required [sic] to be a special Protestant, Catholic, etc., and again a Jewish, heathen psychiatrie. Possibly even this may yet be desired. (Griesinger 1867, p. 348)

Griesinger considered religion to be for many (but not all) patients a useful adjunct to their other care. He noted that patients often improved after a visit by the hospital chaplain, and he attributed this outcome less to what the chaplain said than to the length of time the chaplain spent with the patient.

More important still for the development of psychiatric thinking about worldview, especially as it relates to culture, were the writings of W. H. R. Rivers (1864–1922). Rivers was a neurologist, psychologist, and anthropologist whose thought about the role of culture in shaping worldview and perception of disease and healing have had far-reaching influence. Although Rivers is most often remembered for his work on "shell shock" during World War I, his anthropological work was also very significant. A fellow at St. Johns College, Cambridge, during much of his career, Rivers was a careful ethnologist who studied cultures in South Asia and Melanesia. Among his most enduring books is *Medicine, Magic, and Religion*, published posthumously in 1924, which drew together a wide range of observations about the way various cultures understood and treated diseases. He pointed out that in virtually every culture, diseases are understood as being caused by natural factors; by humans, either naturally or through magic; or by supernatural entities. The treatment of disease involved either natural healing or magical healing, and healers could invoke either or both means of healing. Rivers noted that, despite obvious differences, modern medicine could profitably learn from the study of traditional cultures, and his anthropological studies led him to believe that the "mind" played a crucial role in causing and curing disease (Rivers 1924; Young 1995). Building on these foundations, many psychiatrists of the early and mid-twentieth century have drawn from cross-cultural research to inform their work.

Psychiatric Care in Non-Western Settings

Although more economically "globalized" than ever before, culturally the world remains very heterogeneous. As psychiatry has taken root and grown in different cultures, non-Western psychiatrists have adapted secular and culturally foreign North American or European mental health constructs and techniques to their own cultures, to whatever extent possible (Foulks et al. 1995). At the same time, psychiatrists operating in non-Western settings have raised significant questions about the universality of psychiatric diagnoses. In addition, as people from poorer countries migrate to more prosperous countries in Europe and North America, Western psychiatrists increasingly find themselves treating individuals from unfamiliar cultures. Since the Immigration Reform Act of 1965, the urban areas of the United States have become home to immigrants with worldviews closely aligned to those of the Southern

Hemisphere, not only from Africa, but even larger numbers from Latin America and the Caribbean. These new immigrants often bring with them worldviews based on indigenous religions or, more likely, deeply ingrained Pentecostal or conservative Roman Catholic worldviews (Jenkins 2002). The latter finding will be surprising to many clinicians.

The African Example

In most African countries, the health care infrastructure is suboptimal and modern health care for the impoverished inhabitants of the country is minimal or absent. If general medical care is insufficient, formal mental health care is even less adequate. The vast majority of patients with mental disorders receive treatment based on both Western understandings of the psychiatric problem and traditional methods of treatment.

Some have argued that imposing the usual psychiatric diagnostic and treatment constructs on widely varying cultures is not only meaningless, but ultimately harmful, since it teaches non-Westerners to think about their problems in ways that necessitate expensive, Western-style psychotherapeutics and drug treatments that are not now—and may in fact never be— readily available in their societies (Patel 1996; Summerfield 1999). At the same time, traditional approaches are implicitly delegitimized by these constructs, and people may be deprived of the healing effects of their own traditional approaches, rooted as they are in local worldviews.

Traditional and Western cultures differ sharply in the extent to which they see supernatural forces at work in the events of everyday life. In many parts of the world, such as Africa, most people tend to posit dual explanations for illness and catastrophe, one natural and the other supernatural (Mbiti 1991; Ndetei and Vadher 1985; Patel 1995). In light of the frequency with which shamanism, Pentecostal faith healing, and Islamic religious healing are practiced in large sections of the world (Kleinman 1988), the question of whether secular Western psychotherapies are valuable in the wide range of mental health settings worldwide can be raised. Are secular Western talking therapies that are offered in exchange for financial compensation through formalized health care delivery structures in fact preferable to such traditional approaches?

In Africa, the key to understanding traditional advice lies in understanding African traditional religion, which recognizes no distinction between sacred and secular or between the natural and the supernatural. African traditional religion exists in a variety of forms throughout the continent, but it usually involves each of the following elements: belief in a supreme, unknowable creator-deity; respect for ancestors; observance of specific ceremonies at the time of birth, entry into adulthood, marriage, and death; and a belief in the existence and activity of nature spirits and human spirits with whom humans can interact (Mbiti 1969). Even though most sub-Saharan Africans are adherents of Christianity, African traditional religions continue to exert an influence, much like pre-Christian religion in Europe persists in various forms in the industrialized world in the guise of beliefs in ghosts and the influence of Friday the 13th. As a result, African traditional religion remains a significant, although muted, influence on the worldview of most Africans.

In sub-Saharan Africa, as in much of the world, traditional societies are organized around the tribe or clan. Families in difficult situations and individuals who suffer from emotional distress consult tribal elders, since these elders are viewed as the repository of wisdom for the tribal group. Traditional African family structures often differ significantly from Western family structures. In the African context, kinship relations and tribal context are so important that many observers find individual psychotherapy approaches to be therapeutically ineffective and economically wasteful.

In Kenya, traditional healers are common in both rural and urban areas. Good (1987), in a detailed ethnographic study, found that among 80 *waganga* (witch doctors) he surveyed, mental illness or madness headed the list of conditions they viewed themselves best qualified to treat. Half of them viewed mental illness as something they could treat well, far exceeding their confidence in treating conditions such as abdominal problems, general edema, infertility, impotence, bewitchment, or general body pains (Good 1987, p. 224). Westerners frequently do not understand or account for the existence of these very numerous and widely used healers, and they also fail to realize the importance of the supernatural point of view in the conceptualization of mental (and physical) illness in most of the world.

Treating Western Diseases of Non-Western Patients

Since a number of psychiatric disorders have very different manifestations in different cultures, there is considerable debate about the universal validity of psychiatric diagnostic concepts (Patel 1995; Thakker et al. 1999).

Posttraumatic stress disorder (PTSD) is particularly interesting in this regard. Although some psychiatrists and anthropologists have challenged the universal validity of PTSD, those who have worked with people subjected to overwhelming disaster generally recognize that PTSD, or something very much like it, exists cross-culturally. On the other hand, the meanings people attach to their traumatic experiences may diverge significantly. In the West, an industry has grown up around the treatment of PTSD, so that some have wondered whether efforts to treat the psychological manifestations of trauma have at times overshadowed more important aspects of the problem, such as the causes of the trauma (Summerfield 1999).

The following case example illustrates how a non-Westerner can construe a traumatic experience in a way that a North American or European clinician probably would not expect. This example is drawn from recollections of the August 7, 1998, bombing of the American embassy in Nairobi written by Kenyan employees of the U.S. Foreign Service. The recollections were distributed at a ceremony held in 2000 at the United States ambassador's residence in Nairobi to commemorate the second anniversary of the bombing.

> A 38-year-old Kenyan, an office worker who survived the August 7, 1998, terrorist bombing of the American Embassy in Nairobi, wrote the following recollection 2 years after the bombing. This worker had no psychiatric history, had a long history of successful employment before the bombing, and continued to do well in his job afterward, despite his experience in the bombing. He wrote—
>
> Seven has always been a lucky or sacred number and was given to all manner of grouping in the antiquity.
> SEVEN days of creation
> SEVEN wise men
> SEVEN wonders of the world
> SEVEN churches of Asia
> The SEVEN seas
> The city of SEVEN hills is Rome
> The SEVENTH day is the Sabbath ... Just to mention a few.
> I am also associated with some SEVENS; after all I was born on the SEVENTH (7th) day of May. On the SEVENTH day of August, I had an occasion to witness a life-threatening incident from which I have learnt a lot in life.
> On the fateful day of the SEVENTH of August in 1998, we were a staff of SEVEN in my section: [six numbered names follow] 7. Myself, and we all SURVIVED (Note "SURVIVE" is a SEVEN-letter word.) [sic]
> [Several paragraphs follow in which the office worker gave an account of his experience.]
> In hindsight (looking back), what I regret most about the incident is my inability to assist [omitted] whom I found writhing in pain at the staircase and turned away. But most of all, I thank my Lord and all the other friends and colleagues who participated in saving lives or in playing whatever role during and after the incident. Some people also say that you never know how valuable life is until you experience a situation where you've almost lost it, and this I can vouch for personally.
> My friends may continue believing in the LUCKY SEVEN. I do not want to be superstitious, but I will keep asking them why it had to occur on the SEVENTH day of August.

This Kenyan, who is representative of others who recounted their experience of the bombing, did not experience the event in the same way that most Westerners would have experienced it and would probably not respond to an unmodified psychological approach should he develop symptoms of PTSD (which, in fact, he did not develop). His worldview was clearly influenced by religious concepts (e.g., "sacred"), yet it also included nonreligious elements unique to his experience (e.g., "lucky"). Understanding the worldview of such an individual would be crucially important in developing an effective clinical approach.

Contemporary African cultures are, in general, very religious, and individuals from these cultures often view events in the world from a religious point of view (Jenkins 2002, pp. 34–38). For example, the 1994 Rwandan genocide—during which 800,000 people died (approximately 10% of the population of the country)—was a catastrophe that challenged many aspects of the worldview of those involved. In 1995, 82% of the population of Rwanda was Christian, and of the Christians, approximately two-thirds were Roman Catholic and one-third was Protestant (Barrett et al. 2001). This largely Christian populace had great difficulty understanding how a good God could have let such an event happen.

Mrs. M. is a university-educated Rwandese woman who works for one of the several nongovernmental organizations set up in Kigali to offer mental health care services to Rwandans who survived the genocide. In an interview, she described the personal devastation she experienced during and after the genocide. She had been pregnant, and her husband had been traveling outside the country when the genocide began in April 1994. She fled the city with her small child and lived in the Rwandan bush, surviving by eating whatever could be eaten in that setting. She lost 34 of her 73 kg of body weight during this period. After the end of the genocide in July 1994, she was reunited with her husband. Most of her family had been killed, and she was in despair.

A deeply religious Protestant, she was unable to pray to God between April and December 1994. She could not understand why God had not intervened during the genocide. Her husband prayed for several months after his return that God would release her from her despair. She began to feel that there must have been some reason that God spared her, her child, and her (now) newborn baby, and she began to be able to pray again. She continues to be unable to understand why the atrocities happened, but she believes forgiveness is the key to healing from the effects of the genocide. She is troubled that many Rwandese are unable or unwilling to forgive. Many of the perpetrators of the genocide are not sorry for what they did and cannot be prosecuted by the legal system. She notes that although counseling can be helpful for Rwandese who can receive it, most people have no access to counseling. Mrs. M. believes religion and contact with friends and family are far and away the most common ways people deal with their psychological disturbances, but many people are without family members because of the genocide and she believes that no one cares about what will happen to many of the survivors.

For this woman, faith and the empathy of others began to ameliorate her pain. Her religious belief, while shaken, remained fervent, and the support of her faith community helped rebuild her life. However, she believed from her experience that the trauma had a societal dimension and that healing at a level beyond that of the individual was needed in order for the pain of the individual to be lessened. The healing that needed to take place was intimately connected to the history and tribal makeup of her country.

Neither the survivor of the August 7, 1998, embassy bombing in Kenya nor the survivor of the Rwandan genocide developed PTSD symptoms, although many survivors of both catastrophes did develop these symptoms. The cases of these two individuals illustrate the importance of worldview for understanding how such disasters are experienced.

Extant research supports the idea that members of traditional societies do not conceive of their problems as Westerners conceive of them and that they often find the therapies offered by Westerners of questionable benefit. When Bolton (2001), in a sophisticated ethnographic study, asked Rwandan villagers to do a "free listing" of their problems using Kinyarwanda (the local language) to describe their situation, the top problems were 1) poverty (100%); 2) lack of food (98%); 3) lack of people (61%); and 4) suspicion or breakdown of neighborly relations (56%). Thirty-four percent of the respondents mentioned mental trauma as a top problem, compared with the 100% who listed poverty. A Western effort that offered counseling but failed to address issues of poverty and community disharmony would not be successful in this setting.

In some parts of the world, the nature and meaning of depression is also more complicated and nuanced than psychiatry usually understands them to be. Historically, depression has generally been identified as a disease by Western writers, and the idea of depression as a disease predates Christianity in the West. Yet even depression, a condition often viewed as one of the prototypical universal mental illnesses, seems to be strongly influenced by cultural factors (Widiger and Sankis 2000). For example, it is now commonly observed that somatization, rather than psychological despair, is the most common presentation of depression in the world (Isaac et al. 1995; Kirmayer 2001).

A local understanding of depression, although congruent with the host culture, may seem strange or inappropriate to secularized observers. Obeyesekere (1985) observed that behavior that would be labeled as depression by Western psychiatry is strikingly similar to or identical to a normal state of mind of many observant Buddhists in Sri Lanka who view suffering as a fundamental characteristic of human experience and see even happiness as a form of suffering, since it is impermanent. In this context, bereavement and loss provide an opportunity for reflection on suffering and reaffirm for the believer the Buddhist teaching about the meaning of the human condition. Such a view may produce a state of mind that appears, to the uninitiated, to be depression but that is actually a reflection of a particular worldview.

This point of view can be overstated. It is self-evident to most that something like severe depression does indeed exist in a variety of cultures throughout the world and that some sort of individual attention and appropriate medical therapy leads most patients to welcome relief. On the other hand, appreciation of the varieties of worldviews and individual interpretations of meaning does help us as clinicians to respond more helpfully to our patients.

In a study of the mental health effects of the Rwandan genocide in two villages, Bolton (2001) found that among persons with emotional distress who sought help for their problems, most sought help from local leaders, God, and friends. Most people said they consulted no one. Nongovernmental organization relief staff were available to the villagers but were sought out by very few people. Even when psychotherapy is made available in such circumstances, it is frequently not utilized.

Every patient, of course, brings his or her own worldview to therapy, as does every psychiatrist. Looking at psychotherapy with the global mental health picture in mind helps remind us not only that a set of naturalist or secular Western assumptions underpins much of what we do as therapists, but also that these assumptions—which may seem intuitive—are not shared by most of the people in the world, particularly those in traditional cultures. The further afield from North America and Western Europe that we practice psychotherapy or psychiatry, the less likely it is that patients will understand or benefit from commonly used psychotherapeutic techniques. Even educationally based techniques, such as cognitive therapy, rest on assumptions about the validity of constructs such as depression, anxiety, and PTSD that, in the absence of some modification, may not be valid in a number of settings around the globe.

Once we are aware of our own cultural vantage point, we as clinicians have much to offer individuals outside the Western world who often suffer silently with memories of trauma, anxiety symptoms, and depression—in whatever form these conditions take. However, to be most effective, we need to remember what has been learned from psychiatry as it has been practiced in culturally diverse settings. Taking time to understand as much of the patient's culture as possible—especially the patient's views on morality, ultimate destiny, the meaning of life events (e.g., whether they are preordained, a result of fate, a result of luck, etc.), and the nature of family relationships—helps the clinician develop an empathic, therapeutic relationship. In all cultures, such a relationship allows the patient to unfold his or her narrative and facilitates the clinician's understanding of the meaning of the narrative.

Summary

Clinical experience and the existing literature on cross-cultural psychiatry agree on several points about the role of worldview in clinical practice. First, the way people view the world shapes the way they understand their symptoms and, therefore, the way they present their symptoms. Even the most clearly distinguishable, universal psychiatric disorders are profoundly shaped by culture. Fundamental questions remain about the true nature and conceptual status of diagnoses such as depression and PTSD. Second, the psychiatric approach to any particular individual must be informed by an understanding of the person's view of the world, whether the person is a survivor of the Rwandan genocide with nightmares and intrusive memories or an American Pentecostal with depression and family problems. Failure to adequately consider worldview wastes much effort and money. Third, treatment must be shaped by the patient's worldview. Marx and Spray (1972) have shown that patients tend to choose therapists who share their religious perspective. It is undoubtedly true that therapists are also influenced in their choice of patients by the presence of a shared worldview. Presumably, this selection process can result in inadequate mental health care for segments of the population who do not share therapists' worldviews. Keeping the patient's worldview in mind is particularly important if the worldview of the patient diverges significantly from the ever-narrowing "mainstream" worldview of secular culture.

References

Ackerknecht EH: A Short History of Psychiatry, 2nd Edition. Translated by Wolff S. New York, Hafner, 1968

Barrett DB, Kurian GT, Johnson TM: World Christian Encyclopedia: A Comparative Survey of Churches and Religions in the Modern World, 2nd Edition. New York, Oxford University Press, 2001

Bolton P: Local perceptions of the mental health effects of the Rwandan genocide. J Nerv Ment Dis 189:243–248, 2001

Foulks EF, Bland IJ, Shervington D: Psychotherapy across cultures, in American Psychiatric Press Review of Psychiatry, Vol 14. Edited by Oldham JM, Riba MB. Washington, DC, American Psychiatric Press, 1995, pp 511–528

Good CM: Ethnomedical Systems in Africa: Patterns of Traditional Medicine in Rural and Urban Kenya. New York, Guilford, 1987

Griesinger W: Mental Pathology and Therapeutics. Translated by Robertson CL, Rutherford J. London, New Sydenham Society, 1867

Isaac M, Janca A, Burke KC, et al: Medically unexplained somatic symptoms in different cultures: a preliminary report from phase I of the World Health Organization International Study of Somatoform Disorders. Psychother Psychosom 64:88–93, 1995

Jenkins P: The Next Christendom: The Coming of Global Christianity. New York, Oxford University Press, 2002

Kirmayer LJ: Cultural variations in the clinical presentation of depression and anxiety: implications for diagnosis and treatment. J Clin Psychiatry 62 (suppl 13):22–28; discussion 29–30, 2001

Kleinman A: Rethinking Psychiatry: From Cultural Category to Personal Experience. New York, Free Press, 1988

Marx JH, Spray SL: Psychotherapeutic "birds of a feather": social-class status and religio-cultural value homophily in the mental health field. J Health Soc Behav 13:413–428, 1972

Mbiti JS: African Religions and Philosophy, 2nd Revised and Enlarged Edition. Nairobi, Kenya, East African Educational Publishers, 1969

Mbiti JS: Introduction to African Religion, 2nd Edition. Nairobi, Kenya, East African Educational Publishers, 1991

Ndetei DM, Vadher A: Cross-cultural study of religious phenomenology in psychiatric in-patients. Acta Psychiatr Scand 72:59–62, 1985

Obeyesekere G: Depression, Buddhism, and the work of culture in Sri Lanka, in Culture and Depression: Studies in the Anthropology and Cross-Cultural Psychiatry of Affect and Disorder. Edited by Kleinman A, Good B. Berkeley, CA, University of California Press, 1985, pp 134–152

Patel V: Explanatory models of mental illness in sub-Saharan Africa. Soc Sci Med 40:1291–1298, 1995

Patel V: Recognition of common mental disorders in primary care in African countries: should "mental" be dropped? Lancet 347:742–744, 1996

Rivers WHR: Medicine, Magic, and Religion: The Fitz Patrick Lectures Delivered Before the Royal College of Physicians of London in 1915 and 1916. New York, Harcourt Brace, 1924

Summerfield D: A critique of seven assumptions behind psychological trauma programmes in war-affected areas. Soc Sci Med 48:1449–1462, 1999

Thakker J, Ward T, Strongman KT: Mental disorder and cross-cultural psychology: a constructivist perspective. Clin Psychol Rev 19:843–874, 1999

Widiger TA, Sankis LM: Adult psychopathology: issues and controversies. Ann Rev Psychol 51:377–404, 2000

Young A: The Harmony of Illusions: Inventing Post-Traumatic Stress Disorder. Princeton, NJ, Princeton University Press, 1995

Index

Page numbers printed in **boldface** type refer to tables or figures.